Key Topics in Forensic Psychology

Key Topics in Forensic Psychology provides readers with a succinct yet broad overview of Forensic and Investigative Psychology, considering the history, theories, methods used and key topics where it has been of impact. It also considers where the discipline is headed regarding directions for future research and practice.

Written by academics who have also applied their research in practice, this accessible book outlines the development of Forensic Psychology, from psychological advice given to courts, to assessment and treatment of offenders. It also details the development of Investigative Psychology and how this can assist police investigations. Theoretical explanations of crime are provided with the aid of clear case examples. The book covers a broad variety of applied topics including decision making, eyewitness testimony, suspect interviewing, behavioural investigative advice and the nuances involved in assessment and treatment of offenders. Considering seminal research alongside more recent empirical evidence, the book also considers the various research methods used – from utilisation of vast databases to interviews gleaning in-depth, first-hand knowledge from those involved. Importantly the authors explain how this topic overlaps with other fields such as criminology and law and discuss examples of its wider impact on policy and practice. Finally, the authors consider key emerging areas, such as new crime threats, and suggest new directions for research.

Key Topics in Forensic Psychology is the ideal resource for undergraduate and postgraduate students in this field of psychology, as well as the related areas of criminology and law.

Dr Terri Cole is a Principal Academic in Forensic Psychology at Bournemouth University where she set up their masters course in Investigative Forensic Psychology. This is partially based on her experience of working with the National Crime Agency as a Serious Crime Analyst and then Behavioural Investigative Adviser (offender profiler) for a number of years. Her research interests are focussed mainly on serious crimes and violence against women and girls, helping shape predominantly police practice. She has previously published three books on forensic psychology.

Dr Dara Mojtahedi is a Reader (Associate Professor) in Forensic and Investigative Psychology at the University of Huddersfield. His research spans a diverse range of investigative, legal and criminal psychology; however, his primary research interests are focussed on the evaluation and retrieval of eyewitness memory. Dara has consulted and collaborated with multiple police forces around the world and has informed both parliamentary and international government reports.

BPS Key Topics in Psychology
British Psychological Society

Routledge, in partnership with the British Psychological Society (BPS), is pleased to present *BPS Key Topics in Psychology*, a series of short introductory books that focus on a specific field within psychology. Each book is broken down into bitesize chunks to provide a helpful overview of core psychology topics, made clear by a five-part structure: foundations, theories, methodologies, impacts, and emerging areas. Written by active and experienced authors, these essential books encourage students to approach fundamental concepts with confidence and critical thinking.

Books may incorporate student-friendly pedagogies, including tools such as: feature boxes; key terms and definitions; and links to further reading online. Concise yet comprehensive, these books offer a simple and accessible overview of core psychology topics for students looking for a summary of key concepts in the topic, or those new to the area.

Key Topics in Quantitative Research
Paul Christiansen

Key Topics in Coaching Psychology
Rebecca J. Jones and Holly Andrews

Key Topics in Educational Psychology
Lisa Marks Woolfson

For more information about this series, please visit: www.routledge.com/BPS-Key-Topics-in-Psychology/book-series/BPSKTP

"This textbook incorporates real case examples and guidelines for future practice and research, creating a foundation for discussion and potential empirical studies for both undergraduate and post-graduate students. Additionally, its emphasis on employability is vital and frequently overlooked in academic literature."

Louise Almond, *Professor in Investigative and Forensic Psychology, University of Liverpool.*

"Welcome to what I consider a beginner's guide to the fascinating world of forensic psychology and criminology. This book weaves you through the history of this to now. Along the way you will explore key theories under a forensic psychological lens. From undergraduates to interested onlookers, I highly recommend this book to you, which, once finished, will leave you with a bigger appetite to learn more, and increased confidence in this exciting arena. Enjoy!"

Martyn Underhill, MBE, *Ex Policing Crime Commissioner, Dorset (2012–2021); Senior Lecturer in Criminology, Bournemouth University; Parole Board Member England and Wales.*

"In a crowded market, this is a Forensic text I recommend most highly. It provides an excellent addition to the field, offering a comprehensive yet accessible exploration of the latest developments in Forensic Psychology. The book is rich with case studies, practical insights, and contemporary research developments, making it an invaluable resource for both academics and practitioners. Students will also find this a highly useful resource, helping them to consolidate their learning on the topic."

Dominic Willmott, CPsychol, AFBPsS, *Reader (Associate Professor) in Legal and Criminological Psychology, Loughborough University.*

"Comprehensive, current and critical. A brilliant resource for anyone interested in forensic psychology."

Maria Ioannou, BSc, MSc, PhD, C.Psychol, CSci, AFBPsS, FHEA, CMgr MCMI, *Professor of Investigative and Forensic Psychology, University of Huddersfield.*

Key Topics in Forensic Psychology

Terri Cole and
Dara Mojtahedi

Routledge
Taylor & Francis Group

LONDON AND NEW YORK

Designed cover image: Getty Images

First published 2026
by Routledge
4 Park Square, Milton Park, Abingdon, Oxon OX14 4RN

and by Routledge
605 Third Avenue, New York, NY 10158

Routledge is an imprint of the Taylor & Francis Group, an informa business

© 2026 Terri Cole and Dara Mojtahedi

British Library Cataloguing-in-Publication Data
A catalogue record for this book is available from the British Library

ISBN: 9781032555645 (hbk)
ISBN: 9781032551388 (pbk)
ISBN: 9781003431213 (ebk)

DOI: 10.4324/9781003431213

Typeset in Galliard
by Newgen Publishing UK

Access the Support Material: www.routledge.com/9781032555645

Again, I thank those around me for having the patience and giving me the space to write another book. In particular Darren, Mum, Ken, my mates and my extended family who (hopefully) will be glad to have me back. Ultimately, to my wonderful 'kids' Lily and Alfie, part of the next generation who have found their own paths to happiness and success, and who make me proud (virtually ☺) everyday. Terri

To Mitra and Ebrahim, for keeping my path bright. Dara

Contents

Acknowledgements

Firstly, we would both like to acknowledge the many victims-survivors who are at the heart of the criminal justice system. Unfortunately, their pain and suffering are what predicate this work. We also commend the many professionals working in the field – the work can be both physically and emotionally draining, at times frustrating and often unrecognised. Finally, we thank the students and those attempting to enhance their knowledge by reading this book – we need you, in order to drive forward more research, policy and practice. We also extend a special thank you to Professor Emily Glorney and Doctor Caomh Malone for providing their expert feedback on some of the chapters.

Part I

Key Foundations

Chapter 1

What is Forensic Psychology?

Key Points

Forensic psychology is the application of psychology to the legal system.

There are many types of work – for example working with offenders in prison or whilst on probation, assisting victims, or working with the police.

Forensic psychology links closely to other disciplines such as criminology and law.

What is Psychology?

Psychology is the science of mind and behaviour. Historically in the UK psychology could be studied as either a Bachelor of Arts (BA) or a Bachelor of Science (BSc); however, it is now firmly placed within the arena of **social science**. It looks at both similarities and individual differ-

Psychology. The study of mind and behaviour.

Social Science. The study of people, individuals, societies, their behaviours and interactions.

Nature/Nurture Debate. How much someone's personality or behaviour is formed by biology/genes or their experiences/environment.

ences between people (e.g., some people are more intelligent than others), issues such as the **nature/nurture debate** (are we born this way or does our environment and the people around us shape us?),

DOI: 10.4324/9781003431213-2

4 Key Topics in Forensic Psychology

as well as behavioural consistency and change (e.g., I eat *something* everyday; yet sometimes I want salad and other times prefer cake!). Psychology uses different methods of research, teaching students how to test **hypotheses** using quantitative statistical methods to identify relationships (e.g., as people get older do they offend less?); looking for significant differences (e.g., do males offend more than females?); or considering more nuanced qualitative research questions in more depth (e.g., asking offenders to describe in their own words why they commit crime).

Hypothesis (Plural Hypotheses). Testable statement regarding what is predicted in a research study.

Psychology covers many areas regarding how people think, feel and act. Although generally sub-divided for the purposes of teaching as outlined in Table 1.1, many areas overlap – for example whilst a social psychologist may be interested in how people interact with

Table 1.1 Main Sub-disciplines of Psychology.

Sub-discipline	Description	Areas of study include
Social	How behaviour is affected by social context	Relationships Group behaviour Attitudes Prejudice
Developmental	How humans develop through their lifespan	Child development Adolescence Older adults
Biological/ Neurological	How the brain and hormones influence behaviour	Genetic role in disorders Neurobiological basis Effects of drugs
Cognitive	How we think, learn, understand	Memory Reasoning Decision making Perception Language
Clinical and personality	Mental health/illness and psychological problems	Personality disorders Mental illness and health Assessment Treatment

one another in different contexts, a developmental psychologist may recognise this may be dependent upon someone's age, and a clinical psychologist may recognise this could fluctuate dependent on their mental health at the time. For example, when interacting with a teacher, a child may differ in their interaction if they are in class or if bumping into them out of school (based upon the social environment); a child may interact with the teacher differently given the child's age (based on developmental maturity); or they may interact differently depending on their mental health at the time (if they are particularly anxious about something).

What is Forensic Psychology?

We argue that although **forensic psychology** is a sub-discipline of psychology regarding application and work – it merely applies general psychological theories and methods

Forensic Psychology. Psychology of the legal system – predominantly assessment and treatment of suspects/offenders, but also considers offending, and victims.

to a forensic environment. So for example, when attempting to answer the question of why someone commits crime forensic psychology may consider social aspects (do they need money?), developmental aspects (do they grow out of crime when they get a job, family, responsibilities?), biological aspects (do they have reduced activity in the prefrontal cortex of the brain?), cognitive aspects (do they make poor decisions?) or clinical aspects (do they lack empathy for others?). Links between basic psychological theories and their application to underlying causes of offending are further developed in Chapters 3-7.

The **British Psychological Society** also highlights this applied function to certain roles and settings, stating:

British Psychological Society. The representative body for psychology and psychologists in the UK.

Forensic Psychology is the application of psychology with people and organisations connected with the Court, Health or Justice systems. Our aims would include working with people to create more hopeful futures, supporting pathways to safer communities and to assisting people with a range of mental health experiences towards pathways of recovery and reconnection.

Forensic Psychologists work across many settings including, HM Prison and Probation Service, NHS Trusts, secure health services, Children's services, HM Courts & Tribunals, Universities, Social services, Police forces and a range of Government agencies.

BPS Division of Forensic Psychology

What Work do People do?

Forensic is taken from the Latin word 'forensis' or forum – where the courts were held in ancient Rome. Hence early proponents of

Forensic. Scientific methods applied to investigation of crime or relating to court.

forensic psychology focussed upon work psychologists did in court – as outlined in Figure 1.1. Psychologists with expertise in areas which may be of use in trials (e.g., cognitive psychologists

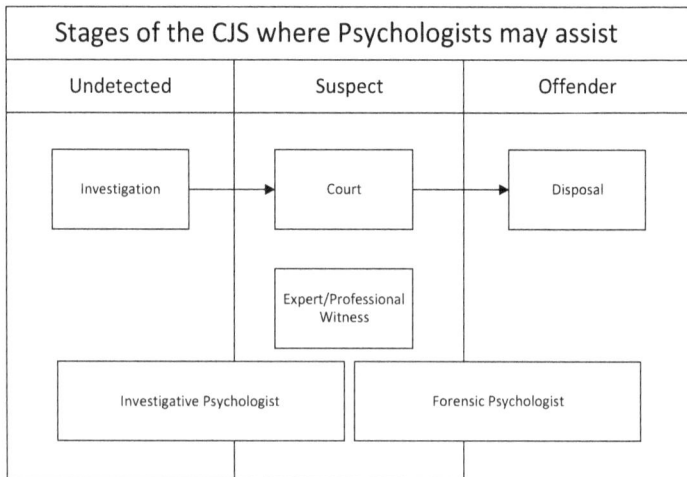

Stages of the CJS where Psychologists may assist

| Undetected | Suspect | Offender |

Investigation → Court → Disposal

Expert/Professional Witness

Investigative Psychologist | Forensic Psychologist

Figure 1.1 Psychologists' input at different stages of the Criminal Justice System.

who had knowledge of memory), provided advice to the court in order to assist juror interpretations and decision making (e.g., in relation to the reliability of eyewitness testimony).

The discipline then developed as is outlined in greater detail in Chapter 2, with forensic psychologists assessing individuals to determine whether they were fit to stand trial and if incarcerated, which **disposal** (prison or hospital) would be most appropriate. Moreover, psychologists then became involved in treatment of offenders (see Chapter 15) and in assessing and reducing the risk they pose to themselves and others (see Chapter 14), for

Disposal. The sentence or outcome of a case.

Forensic Psychologist. Assesses criminal behaviour and helps people who have committed crimes. A protected title – i.e., can only be used by someone with specific qualifications.

example indicating to parole boards whether or not they felt offenders were ready for release back into society from prison or a secure hospital. This role of a **forensic psychologist** involves "*working with people… to help them address factors associated with risk of further offending and develop healthy, prosocial lives*" (British Psychological Society, n.d.). As such the focus for many forensic psychologists working in prisons, secure hospitals, in community forensic services or with those on probation, is still very much based on working with offenders and the reduction of future offending.

More recently psychologists have been assisting law enforcement, initially as occupational psychologists in areas such as recruitment, promotion and retention; or in more therapeutic roles for example providing support to police officers working undercover or in debriefing traumatic cases on which they may have worked. A newer sub-discipline of **investigative psychology** to assist police investigations,

Investigative Psychology. Application of psychology to the criminal investigation process.

identifying and helping bring offenders to justice is now firmly established alongside traditional roles, with bespoke courses and employment focussing on these areas.

Hence the work of psychologists has developed and expanded over time. It began in the 'middle' of the **criminal justice system** in the courts, moved to the 'latter end' working with offenders and patients in relation to disposal, and now also includes the 'early stages' of the criminal justice system, being involved in attempting to identify offenders, analysing patterns of crimes and advising on matters such as police interviewing techniques. Underpinning all of this work has been research, examples of which are provided throughout this book. As seen in Figure 1.1, psychologists now input at all stages of the criminal justice system – with investigative psychologists focussing more on the period from the crime occurring to identifying and bringing suspects to court, and more traditional forensic psychologists focussing on assisting court decisions, and in considering the risk, treatment and management of offenders post-charge or conviction.

Criminal Justice System. Collection of agencies related to bringing criminals to justice including police, courts, prison and probation.

How Does Forensic Psychology Link to Other Disciplines?

As discussed above, psychology focusses on behaviour, and therefore forensic and investigative psychologists consider interactions between offender and victim, motivations, decisions and background factors. However, some of these overlap with other disciplines, as neatly summarised by Clive Hollin:

> *Academics like nothing better than dividing the world into discrete disciplines in an attempt to bring order into our everyday lives. However, some topics irritatingly refuse to fall into line… leaving several disciplines laying claim to a particular area. This point is particularly true when it comes to crime.*
>
> taken from Brown, Shell & Cole (2015, p324)

In addition, in practice it is impossible to work in a silo. Multidisciplinary working is now the norm. At a crime scene a psychologist may be working with a forensic scientist and detective; in a secure hospital a psychologist may be working with a psychiatrist or nurse, and in court a psychologist will be liaising with a **lawyer**.

Moreover, it is necessary to have an understanding of the end goal of your work and the related legislation, rules and regulations **Lawyer.** Person licensed to advise about law or represent clients in court e.g., solicitor, barrister.

when performing your role. A psychologist advising police in relation to an interview strategy must have at least some knowledge of the Police and Criminal Evidence Act[1], rules of disclosure[2] and PEACE interviewing[3] practice for example, otherwise the advice they provide could be invalid at best, but even worse unethical, misleading or counter-productive (see Box 11.4). Similarly, if giving evidence in court a forensic psychologist needs to understand the different courts, roles within them and different types of witness (e.g., whether they have been called as either a professional or expert witness would have a bearing on whether or not they are able to offer an opinion). Whilst some basic knowledge and a level of mutual respect of other disciplines and roles is essential, it is not without difficulties. Eastman (2000) used the analogy of 'Legaland' and 'Mentaland' to explain two different 'countries' lawyers and psychologists could come from – each with its own history, language and culture, which at times are incongruous. Each 'country' has different methods and priorities – for example a psychologist is an objective scientist, whereas a lawyer is paid to represent one side. Hence there is a need to be cognisant of the conflicts which are likely to occur within and between professions, and understand how differences in disciplines and focus may lead to confusion and contradiction, if not carefully considered (for a more detailed discussion of these similarities and differences see Ogloff & Finkelman, 1999). Some of the main disciplines related to forensic psychology are outlined in Figure 1.2.

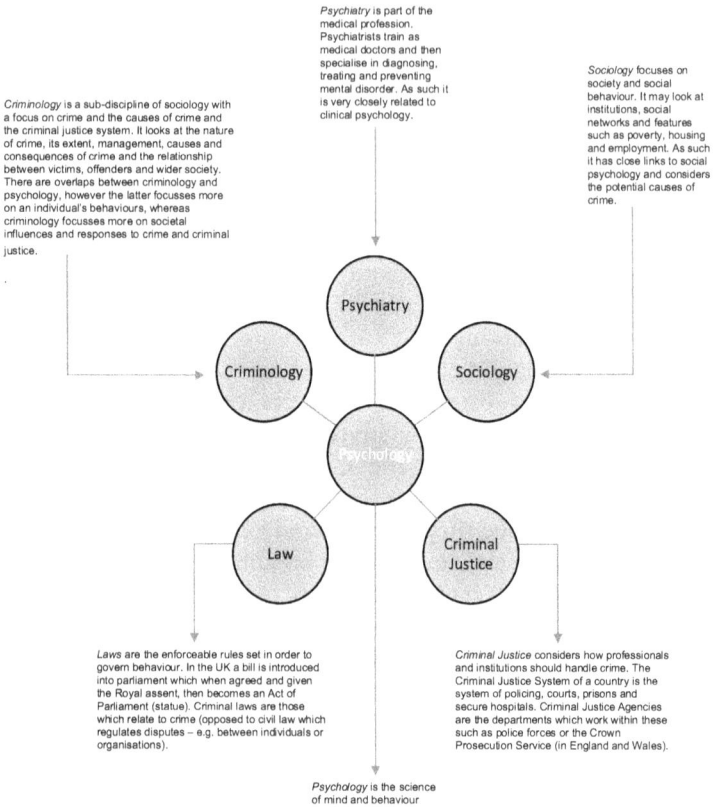

Psychiatry is part of the medical profession. Psychiatrists train as medical doctors and then specialise in diagnosing, treating and preventing mental disorder. As such it is very closely related to clinical psychology.

Sociology focuses on society and social behaviour. It may look at institutions, social networks and features such as poverty, housing and employment. As such it has close links to social psychology and considers the potential causes of crime.

Criminology is a sub-discipline of sociology with a focus on crime and the causes of crime and the criminal justice system. It looks at the nature of crime, its extent, management, causes and consequences of crime and the relationship between victims, offenders and wider society. There are overlaps between criminology and psychology, however the latter focusses more on an individual's behaviours, whereas criminology focusses more on societal influences and responses to crime and criminal justice.

Psychiatry

Criminology

Sociology

Psychology

Law

Criminal Justice

Laws are the enforceable rules set in order to govern behaviour. In the UK a bill is introduced into parliament which when agreed and given the Royal assent, then becomes an Act of Parliament (statue). Criminal laws are those which relate to crime (opposed to civil law which regulates disputes – e.g. between individuals or organisations).

Criminal Justice considers how professionals and institutions should handle crime. The Criminal Justice System of a country is the system of policing, courts, prisons and secure hospitals. Criminal Justice Agencies are the departments which work within these such as police forces or the Crown Prosecution Service (in England and Wales).

Psychology is the science of mind and behaviour

Figure 1.2

Outline of this Book

Although the focus of the book is narrative yet academic, it is provided as a summary of each topic. Wider reading can be enjoyed via searches for recent journal articles, or through the further reading links; however, this book gives a basic grounding on theories, methods, and impacts the discipline has made, is currently making or, in the final chapters, aspirations we hope it makes in future. Chapters are short and designed to be easy to read; the book can be read as a whole, or chapters can stand alone for interest in specific areas (cross references to other chapters are made where appropriate). Interspersed are boxes with examples, commentary, key cases and ideas to bring to life some of the points raised – and to break the monologue of purely academic text! We have also included anecdotes and analogies to everyday life in recognition of the fact that learning is best embedded within notions with which we are already familiar.

Chapter 2 continues this discussion on key foundations, considering the historical development of forensic psychology from early research and practice, and expanding upon how forensic and investigative psychology are applied and studied today.

Chapters 3–7 consider some of the key theories in relation to why people may commit crime. These detail theories from psychology and the related disciplines explored above in relation to cognitive, developmental, social and situational, neurological, personality and clinical psychology.

Chapters 8 and 9 consider some of the key methods used in psychology, presenting examples of both quantitative and qualitative methods, and how they have been used in some of our own forensic and investigative research.

Chapters 10–15 consider bespoke areas and key impacts that forensic and investigative psychology have made in relation to research, policy and practice. Chapter 10 discusses witness evidence considering features such as memory conformity and weapon focus effect. Chapter 11 focuses upon behavioural analysis of crimes – discussing the work of different crime analysts and Behavioural Investigative Advisers. Chapter 12 considers the impact psychology has had in relation to interviewing suspects comparing interrogative and investigative interviewing approaches. Chapter 13 focuses on the difficult task of investigative decision making which often occurs in high stake, fast paced environments. Chapters 14 and 15 describe the role of psychologists in assessing and attempting to treat and manage offenders. It considers the debate of 'what works' (if anything) in reducing risk of reoffending (recidivism) and enhancing future lives.

The final two chapters consider current topics of interest and look forward, to consider future areas of research in Chapter 16, and potential implications for policy and practice in Chapter 17. Although the chapters are separated, roles of academics and practitioners in forensic and investigative psychology are increasingly merged, with academics advising practise and undertaking research designed to impact society; and practitioners increasingly recognising the need for co-creating evidence-based research with academics or undertaking it themselves. As an applied discipline, most people join the profession to make a difference of some kind – to scientific theory, to society, to individuals and ultimately to understand and reduce criminality and suffering. How psychology undertakes this unenviable task, is the focus of this book.

Notes

1 Police and Criminal Evidence Act 1984 (legislation.gov.uk)
2 Disclosure – The Crown Prosecution Service (cps.gov.uk)
3 Investigative interviewing – College of Policing (college.police.uk)

Further Reading

Video – This video considers what is Forensic Psychology? www.youtube.com/watch?v=HMPIvOUvqPA

Web pages – The British Psychological Society website has a specific area for Forensic Psychology which includes videos and useful information – bps.org.uk/member networks/division-forensic-psychology

UK legislation is published and searchable – legislation.gov.uk

The Crown Prosecution website is also a great source for legal documents – cps.gov.uk

The College of Policing UK is also a very good source for policing guidance – college.police.uk

Podcasts – "Let's Talk Forensic Psychology" and "the Forensic Psychology Podcast" utilise experience of many working in the field and detail general work for example within the HM Prison and Probation Service.

References

British Psychological Society (n.d.). *DFP*. Retrieved February 18, 2025, from www.bps.org.uk/member networks/division-forensic-psychology

Brown, J., Shell, Y., & Cole, T. (2015). *Forensic psychology: Theory, research, policy and practice.* Sage.

Eastman, N. L. G. (2000). Psycholegal studies as an interface discipline. In J. McGuire, T. Mason, & A. O'Kane, (Eds.), *Behaviour, Crime and Legal Processes: A Guide for Forensic Practitioners.*

Ogloff, J. R. P., & Finkelman, D. (1999). Psychology and law. In R. Roesch, S. D. Hart & J. R. P. Ogloff, (Eds.), *Psychology and law. Perspectives in law & psychology*, vol 10. Springer. https://doi.org/10.1007/978-1-4615-4891-1_1

Chapter 2

Early Beginnings and Development of Forensic Psychology

Key Points

Early psychological research began with laboratory experiments and empiricism.
Psychology then became more applied and developed into a specific profession.
Practice developed over time to include the use of psychology in court, for assessment and treatment of offenders, and assisting investigations.

Early Research

1879: Wilhelm Wundt has been labelled as the 'first' psychologist – the 'father' of psychology, owing to his founding the first psychological laboratory in Leipzig, Germany in 1879, advocating the use of **experimental methods** and approaches. Some of this early research investigated conscious experience – getting participants to verbalise to the researcher external feelings (**introspection**) such as sensation, and internal thoughts such as perception. Other research methods were more experimental, akin to more traditional forms of science within the laboratory – but rather

Experimental Methods. Systematic procedures/steps to gather data and analyse results.
Introspection. Examination of one's own thoughts and feelings.

DOI: 10.4324/9781003431213-3

than mixing chemicals to test reactions, recorded observations of human behaviours such as reaction time (see Wundt, 1948).

1894: Studying under Wundt, James Cattell developed **psychological testing** – as an early proponent of applied psychology, he promoted its use in real-world settings. For example, testing memories of everyday life (e.g., the weather the previous week) rather than testing memories of numbers/letters. He found great variation in responses and whilst recall could be poor, participants could appear overly confident – not remembering well, yet thought they did. This has obvious implications when relying upon crime statements – witnesses may inaccurately recall information yet give evidence with confidence in court.

> **Psychological Testing**. Instruments to measure behavioural characteristics – for example personality.

1908: Another protégé of Wundt, Hugo Munsterberg published 'On the Witness Stand' commenting in its introduction:

> *Experimental psychology has reached a stage at which it seems natural and sound to give attention also to its possible service for the practical needs of life…. to adjust research to the practical problems themselves.*
>
> Munsterberg, 1908, p8–9.

He demonstrated the potential usefulness of psychology in court for legal matters including the accuracy of witnesses' memory, why people may falsely confess to crimes, what influences suggestibility, crime prevention and how jurors make decisions regarding guilt or innocence.

1916: Lewis Terman (Terman et al., 1917) initially applied psychology to policing by creating **intelligence** and **aptitude tests** for military and law enforcement, to

> **Intelligence Tests**. Tests to identify and quantify cognitive abilities e.g., verbal, maths.
> **Aptitude Tests**. Tests to identify level of skill or ability to succeed at a given activity.

screen and choose the best candidates with relevant traits and abilities for particular jobs.

1917: A year later William Marston began experiments attempting to detect deception. He found when people were known to be lying their blood pressure increased, which led to the creation of an early form of a lie detector (**polygraph**). Although the use of such tests are somewhat controversial and more reliable measures have subsequently been developed (e.g., Vrij, Fisher & Blank, 2017), these methods are still used in some areas. For example, the probation service in England and Wales use polygraph testing to monitor high risk sex offenders (and more recently domestic abuse offenders[1]) to enhance self-reported offending (for discussion see Grubin, 2016).

Polygraph. Machine which detects physiological changes – used in lie detection.

1939: William Stern highlighted:

> *Perfectly correct remembrance is not the rule but the exception; that even the most favourable conditions for witnessing and remembering fail to protect people against illusions.*
>
> Stern, 1939, p3.

Memory has been a core topic of psychology considering what, how, in what circumstances and when people remember. Importantly what situations can enhance, or hinder encoding, retrieval and accuracy have been applied for example in relation to appropriate questioning techniques for investigative interviewing. Stern found emotions could impact on memory, thus affecting how and what potentially traumatised eyewitnesses to crimes may recall. Stern also found memory declined over time – hence his work had implications for when statements from witnesses were taken (the sooner after the event, the better) and how verbal evidence in court is prompted and recalled.

As such, psychology grew from the utilisation of experimental methods in a laboratory, to **empiricism**

Empiricism. Knowledge comes from evidence via sensory experience or observations.

with the scientific approach of generating hypotheses, gathering **data** and evidence to repeatedly test them, and creating **theories** to assist in prediction of future events. With

Data. Any information that is collected or measured – for example words, measures.
Theories. Ideas to explain something.

enhanced knowledge, and an increasing willingness to apply this to real world environments, testify in courts, assist in trial preparation and jury selection (in the USA) – the sub-discipline of forensic psychology developed.

Development of the Profession

McGuire and Duff (2018) note that in 1887 not only did the academic publication 'American Journal of Psychology' begin to share psychological knowledge, but also the first independent psychology department was established (at Clark University). The American Psychological Society – a formal organisation recognising the work of psychologists – was created in 1892, and shortly after, in 1901, the British Psychological Society (BPS) was formed.

Forensic Psychology was recognised as a specialism by the BPS in 1999 (with a Division of Legal and Criminological Psychology set up in 1977); and by the **American Psychological Association** (APA) in 2001 (Brown, 2015). This was closely followed by the development of standard practice, regulations (e.g., by the **Health and Care Professions Council** in 2010) and formal assessments of competency

American Psychological Association. The professional organisation representing psychologists in the USA.
Health and Care Professions Council. Regulator of all health and care professions in the UK – for example sets standards and keeps a register of professionals.

and accreditation. Interested candidates should note there are significant requirements to become a 'forensic psychologist[2]', (which do not currently exist to work in the more investigative fields).

Since then, there has been a proliferation of specialist under-graduate and post-graduate courses all over the world, with researchers exploring a variety of topics, and new roles expanding for psychology practitioners within forensic and related domains.

Development of Practice

We argued in Chapter 1 that forensic psychology developed from initial court testimony; to recognition and assessment of mental illness and treatment of offenders; and more latterly to assisting investigations.

Court

Early definitions of forensic psychology highlighted its use as evidence assisting judicial or legal decisions (Blackburn, 1996; Haward, 1981). The first recorded **expert psychological testimony** was in 1896 by another student of Wundt, Albert von Schrenk-Notzing. In support of a man convicted of murder, he used research in relation to suggestibility, to highlight the potential influence of pre-trail publicity. He argued witnesses may be unable to distinguish what they had read in the press – uncorroborated and potentially unreliable hearsay; and what had actually been witnessed in court – the only information which should be considered in consideration of guilt or innocence. Such 'post-event misinformation' has been widely researched and its implications are still recognised today (see Chapter 10).

Gavin (2019) summarises that although insanity was not deemed a **mitigating factor** in English law

Expert (Psychological) Testimony. Expert opinion provided by a qualified individual to provide the court with information outside the experience and knowledge of the judge/jury.

Mitigating Factors. Factors which may reduce the seriousness of the crime or severity of the sentence – e.g., admitting an offence, provocation or showing remorse.

until the fourteenth century, back in 340 BC Aristotle theorised a person should only be responsible for a crime if he had knowledge of the circumstances and acted without compulsion (impulse). In 1723 if someone did not understand what they were doing was wrong (akin to an infant or 'wild beast') they were exempt from punishment. Legal decisions considering state of mind in relation to intent (e.g., murder) or whether actions were merely reckless or neglectful (e.g., manslaughter), can be enhanced by psychological research or evaluation. For example, a train driver could be mitigated for crashing into something on a train line, if it could be demonstrated any reasonable person would not have had time to react.

Today psychologists can assist the court in a variety of instances, for example, research in relation to the behaviour of rape or domestic violence victims can inform jurors; diagnoses from clinical or forensic psychologists can influence decisions surrounding a suspect's **fitness to plead** or the appropriate disposal for a convicted offender (prison or hospital). Extension has been made from the criminal courtroom to application of psychological knowledge and expertise in other legal hearings including the **family court**, **appeal courts**, **mental health tribunals** or boards discussing eligibility for **parole** (McGuire & Duff, 2018).

Fitness to Plead (USA – Competence to Stand Trial). The capacity of a defendant to comprehend court proceedings.

Family Court. Decides matters in relation to family law – for example custody of children.

Appeal Courts. Deal with appeals from other courts –against conviction or sentence.

Mental Health Tribunals. Panels to hear applications from those who have had their liberty restricted under the Mental Health Act – e.g., have been sectioned.

Parole (Boards). Determine if prisoners can be safely released.

Assessment and treatment of offenders

Practice then developed further into looking at assessment and treatment of individuals. As is discussed in Chapter 14, assessments continue throughout the criminal justice process – for example suspects are assessed as to whether they are fit to stand trial, offenders are assessed when receiving a custodial sentence to see where they should be detained (prison or hospital); and subsequently assessed as to whether they are ready for release. Assessments are also undertaken to formulate a treatment plan for the offender if required (and available[3]).

Treatment – predominantly trying to change behaviour and enhance the likelihood they will desist from crime, is the focus of much practice (see Chapter 15). What (if anything) works, whether intervention should take place, when, and in what form – are key debates. McGuire and Duff (2018) attribute the first use of treatment recommendations to juvenile offenders to Healy who in 1909 founded an institute in Chicago which assessed and suggested treatment recommendations to courts in relation to juvenile offenders. By 1918 the first inmate classification system was developed in New Jersey to:

> *Provide programs and environments for offenders designed to effect changes in behaviour …to assess the personality and needs … and equip the offender to function in a positive, self-fulfilling manner in society after release.*
>
> Hippchen, 1975

In 1924 Wisconsin became the first state to offer psychological examinations to all those entering the prison system or applying for parole (Bartol & Bartol, 2015).

As noted by Brown (2015) in her engaging collection of seminal research articles charting the development of Forensic Psychology, by the 1970's clearer definitions of roles and contexts in which Forensic Psychologists could work had been created. For example, by 1972 'correctional' psychology (i.e., for those working with offenders) became recognised as a professional career (Bartol & Bartol, 2015).

Psychologists working in this field today collect information about an individual's behaviour and experiences to reduce (via management and treatment) future harm they may cause to others, or themselves (McGuire & Duff, 2018).

Assisting investigations

The link between psychology and policing became increasingly apparent during the 1970's when changes in mental health provision – closing many inpatient facilities, instead providing 'care in the community'; meant law enforcement were often the first to deal with individuals experiencing crisis (Massey, 2015). Yet as noted in the previous chapter, the development of psychology in policing began traditionally from other fields such as occupational psychology concerned with recruitment, welfare concerns for those deployed under cover or on traumatic cases, and latterly into practically offering advice, research and analysis to policing practice.

As is further explored in Chapter 10, early utility came in the form of offering advice to gain witness evidence. Methods incorporated into police practice include how best to reliably obtain identification evidence (see Pike & Clark, 2018) and more recently use of '**super recognisers**' in identification of offenders from CCTV evidence for example (see Davis & Robertson, 2020; Portch et al., 2024). Use of techniques for retrieval of information from interviews has also been widely explored. For example, utilisation of '**cognitive interviews**' for compliant witnesses was developed, tested and is now widely used (Fisher et al., 1989) and subsequently techniques suggested how to interview those less willing or able to engage (Wells & Brandon, 2019). Also, work in relation to **suggestibility** (Gudjonsson, 1984), for example considering variables which may lead suspects to falsely confess to crimes they have not committed, and more general methods of detecting deception (Vrij et al., 2022) have been examined.

> **Super Recognisers**. People with better than average face recognition abilities.
> **Cognitive Interview**. Questioning technique used to enhance retrieval of information.
> **Suggestibility**. Being inclined to accept suggestions of others e.g., in police interviews.

In terms of assisting the investigative process, the usefulness of pragmatic decision making has been recognised (Alison et al., 2007; Ask & Fahsing, 2019). To assist with investigator decision making and prioritisation of resources, investigative agencies have developed bespoke roles of Researchers, Crime Analysts, Geographic Profilers and Behavioural Investigative Advisers. In various guises these professionals help in summarising offence patterns and prioritising areas or potential persons of interest (see Chapter 11).

Summary

As indicated above, from psychological experiments in a laboratory, to applying theories initially to court, and then incorporating practice into wider criminal justice settings such as prisons and policing; forensic and investigative psychology developed. The scientific approach of gathering data to test hypotheses, and developing and applying theories led to the development of the profession of forensic psychology.

Notes

1 A useful polygraph test factsheet can be found here: www.gov.uk/gov ernment/publications/domestic-abuse-bill-2020-factsheets/mandat ory-polygraph-tests-factsheet
2 British Psychological Society qualifications can be found here: www. bps.org.uk/bps-qualifications; the APA guide of how to become a psychologist can be found here: www.apa.org/education-career/ guide; requirements for getting onto the Health and Care Professions Council register can be found here: www.hcpc-uk.org/registration/ getting-on-the-register/
3 Often only certain offenders (e.g., high risk) or with recognisable, potentially 'manageable' traits (e.g., anger) are offered treatment.

Further Reading

Books – In addition to the reference list below an enlightening four volume collection of key historical writings, and the foundational works of the critical concepts in forensic psychology has been compiled by Professor Jennifer Brown. Brown, J. (2015) *Forensic Psychology. Critical Concepts in Psychology.* Routledge.

Video – This website contains a video with information regarding the Health and Care Professions Council www.hcpc-uk.org

Web pages – The classic book by Hugo Munsterberg, including discussion of his famous 'clown in a conference' study highlighting the fallibility of memory (p51–52) is replicated here https://jscholarship.libr ary.jhu.edu/bitstream/1774.2/33579/302/31151024684734.pdf

Podcasts – "Forensic Psychology Careers" detail the potential application and careers including for example work of those in prison, probation, mental health, in the police and undertaking research.

References

Alison, P. L., Barrett, E., & Crego, J. (2007). Criminal investigative decision making: Context and process. In R. R. Hoffman (Ed.), *Expertise out of context* (pp. 86–102). Psychology Press. https://doi.org/10.4324/9780203810088

Ask, K., & Fahsing, I. (2019). Investigative decision making. In R. Bull & I. Blandón-Gitlin (Eds.), *The Routledge International handbook of legal and investigative psychology* (pp. 84–101). Routledge. https://doi.org/10.4324/9780429326530

Bartol, C. R., & Bartol, A. M. (2015). *Introduction to forensic psychology: Research and application.* Sage.

Blackburn, R. (1996). What is forensic psychology?. *Legal and Criminological Psychology, 1*(1), 3–16.

Brown, J. (2015). *Forensic psychology. Critical concepts in psychology.* Routledge.

Davis, J., & Robertson, D. (2020). Capitalizing on the super-recognition advantage: A powerful, but underutilized, tool for policing and national security agencies. *Journal of the Homeland Defense & Security Information Analysis Centre, 7*(1), 20–25.

Fisher, R. P., Geiselman, R. E., & Amador, M. (1989). Field test of the Cognitive Interview: Enhancing the recollection of actual victims and witnesses of crime. *Journal of Applied Psychology, 74*(5), 722.

Gavin, H. (2019). *Criminological and forensic psychology.* Sage.

Grubin, D. (2016). Treatment of sex offenders: Strengths and weaknesses in assessment and intervention. Polygraph testing of sex offenders. *Polygraph, 45,* 97.

Gudjonsson, G. H. (1984). A new scale of interrogative suggestibility. *Personality and Individual Differences, 5*(3), 303–314.

Haward, L. R. C. (1981). Expert opinion based on evidence from forensic hypnosis and lie-detection. In S. M. A. Lloyd-Bostock (Ed.), *Psychology in legal contexts.* Oxford Socio-Legal Studies. Palgrave Macmillan. https://doi.org/10.1007/978-1-349-04917-2_8

Hippchen, J. (1975). The basis for modern treatment of offenders. *Office of Justice Partners.* Retrieved March 10, 2025, from www.ojp.gov/ncjrs/virtual-library/abstracts/classification-basis-modern-treatment-offenders-correctional

Massey, K. (2015). Policing and mental health. In M. Brunger, S. Tong & D. Martin (Eds.), *Introduction to policing research* (pp. 57–70). Routledge.

McGuire, J., & Duff, S. (2018). *Forensic psychology: Routes through the system.* Bloomsbury.

Münsterberg H. (1908). *On the witness stand: Essays in psychology and crime.* Doubleday, Page. https://doi.org/10.1037/10854-000

Pike, G., & Clark, C. (2018). Identification evidence. In A. Griffiths & R. Milne (Eds.), *The psychology of criminal investigation* (pp. 133–153). Routledge.

Portch, E., Attard-Johnson, J., Estudillo, A. J., Mestry, N., & Bate, S. (2024). "Super-recognizers" and the legal system. In E. Pica, D. Ross & J. Pozzulo (Eds.), *The impact of technology on the criminal justice system* (pp. 272–300). Routledge.

Stern, W. (1939). The psychology of testimony. *The Journal of Abnormal and Social Psychology*, *34*(1), 3–20. https://doi.org/10.1037/h0054144

Terman, L. M., Otis, A. S., Dickson, V., Hubbard, O. S., Norton, J. K., Howard, L., & Cassingham, C. C. (1917). A trial of mental and pedagogical tests in a civil service examination for policemen and firemen. *Journal of Applied Psychology*, *1*(1), 17–29. https://doi.org/10.1037/h0073841

Vrij, A., Fisher, R. P., & Blank, H. (2017). A cognitive approach to lie detection: A meta-analysis. *Legal Criminal Psychology*, *22*, 1–21. https://doi.org/10.1111/lcrp.12088

Vrij, A., Granhag, P. A., Ashkenazi, T., Ganis, G., Leal, S., & Fisher, R. P. (2022). Verbal lie detection: Its past, present and future. *Brain Sciences*, *12*(12), 1644.

Wells, S., & Brandon, S. E. (2019). Interviewing in criminal and intelligence-gathering contexts: Applying science. *International Journal of Forensic Mental Health*, *18*(1), 50–65.

Wundt, W. (1948). *Principles of physiological psychology.* Retrieved March 10, 2025, from http://elibrary.bsu.edu.az/files/books_163/N_152.pdf

Part II

Key Theories

Chapter 3

Cognitive Theories of Crime

Key Points

Cognitive Neoassociation Theory and the General Aggression Model explain how the appraisal of an aversive incident can lead to reactive aggression. The latter model considers how individual differences, and situational factors interact during aggressive episodes.

Cognitive distortions are biased patterns of thinking which can promote maladaptive/criminal behaviours. Certain offending groups have distorted views of the world.

Understanding the cognitive processes that underpin criminal behaviour alongside maladaptive behaviour patterns that promote offending can inform strategies that target crime prevention.

Understanding the cognitive processes that underpin criminal behaviour, by for example identifying maladaptive patterns of thinking (**cognitive distortions**) can elucidate how individuals arrive at the decision to offend and can also inform rehabilitative strategies. This chapter draws on cognitive theories to explain mental processes that precede criminal behaviour.

Cognitive Distortions. Biased thoughts that distort the way an individual perceives themselves and/or others. Can promote maladaptive behaviour.

DOI: 10.4324/9781003431213-5

Firstly, we explore the cognitive processes underpinning aggression in violent crime, followed by an examination of different thinking patterns promoting criminal activity more generally.

Cognitive Models of Aggression and Violence

Cognitive Neoassociation (CNA) Theory

Individual differences in violent behaviour can be explained by variations in how individuals appraise and emotionally react to actions of others (Berkowitz, 1990). The **Cognitive Neoassociation (CNA) theory** (Berkowitz, 1989, 2008) builds on earlier models of reactive aggression (e.g., the **Frustration-Aggression Hypothesis**) adding consideration of the relationship between negative affect (feeling) and cognitive appraisal (thinking).

Cognitive Neoassociation Theory. Reactive aggression is a product of the cognitive processing of negative affect following an aversive incident.

Frustration-Aggression Hypothesis. Early theory that frustration leads to aggressive behaviour.

According to CNA (illustrated in Figure 3.1), an aversive event can produce a negative effect, which is instinctively, unconsciously and immediately processed, triggering a fight or flight reaction. Fight impulses activate thoughts, memories and physiological/motor reactions related to aggression; whereas flight impulses activate reactions to escape danger.

The individual will then consciously appraise these rudimentary emotions in conjunction with the initial incident, outcome expectations and social rules, and consolidates these into a "collection of particular feelings, expressive motor reactions, thoughts, and memories that are associated" Berkowitz (1993, p. 59). Although the CNA stops at the internal state of consolidated emotion, it is implied that flight stems from fear, whereas aggressive behaviours stem from consolidated feelings of irritation, annoyance or anger (Berkowitz, 2012).

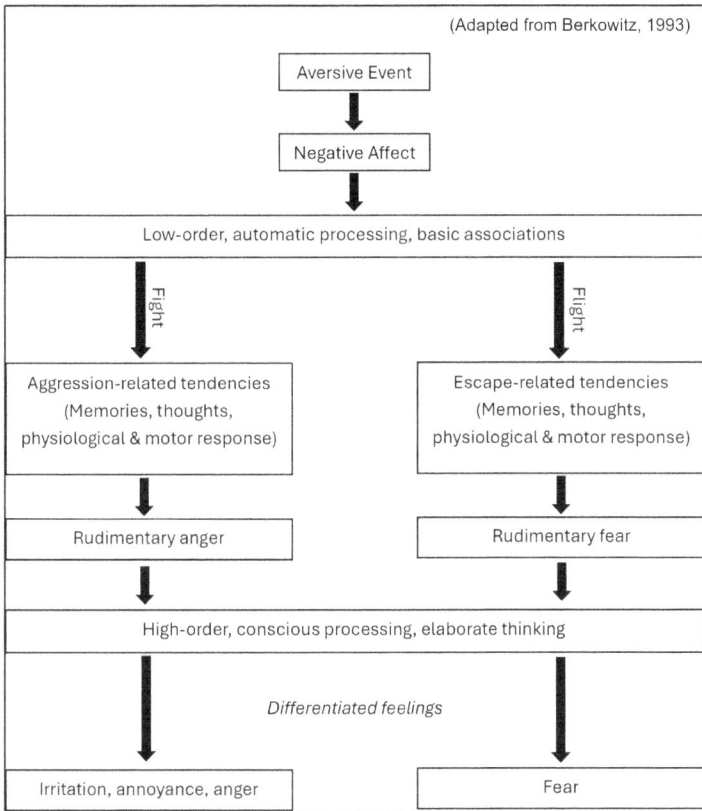

(Adapted from Berkowitz, 1993)

Aversive Event

↓

Negative Affect

↓

Low-order, automatic processing, basic associations

Fight

Flight

Aggression-related tendencies
(Memories, thoughts,
physiological & motor response)

Escape-related tendencies
(Memories, thoughts,
physiological & motor response)

↓

↓

Rudimentary anger

Rudimentary fear

↓

↓

High-order, conscious processing, elaborate thinking

Differentiated feelings

↓

↓

Irritation, annoyance, anger

Fear

Figure 3.1 Visual representation of the Cognitive Neoassociation Model.

General Aggression Model (Anderson & Bushman, 2002)

The CNA advanced understanding of aggression; however, the theory does not consider the impact of personality and past experiences, nor recognise the interplay between learning, mental representation and interpretations of social cues (Fiske, 2009). An integrative model was developed by Anderson and Bushman to integrate social learning (Bandura, 2001), script theory (Huesmann, 1986), excitation transfer theory (Zillmann & Bryant, 1974) and CNA (Berkowitz, 1989) – the **General Aggression Model** (GAM; Anderson & Bushman, 2002). This model considers how inherent dispositions (e.g., genetics, neurological factors and upbringing), the development and mainten-

General Aggression Model. An integrative model of aggression that shows how how distal processes (internal characteristics) interact with proximate processes (social interaction and cognitive appraisal) to influence aggression.

ance of aggression-related knowledge structures (e.g., attitudes, beliefs, cognitive biases), and environmental factors interact to inform aggressive outcomes.

The GAM is represented as two interconnected components that precede aggressive behaviour (see Figure 3.2). *Distal processes* represent inherent traits (i.e., personality) that enable aggression within social situations. Such traits are shaped over time through both biological (e.g., genetics and neurological factors (see Chapter 6) and environmental modifiers (e.g., childhood experiences and social interactions in adulthood). These factors can work in isolation or interact to yield individual differences in aggressive dispositions. *Proximate processes* represent the situational elements that precede aggressive reactions. This stems from the initial interaction between the individual and a situation (trigger). Both elements link back to personality traits which not only inform an individual's susceptibility to aggression but also their probability of encountering aggressive situations. Interaction between a situational trigger and the self will evoke interrelated cognitions, emotions and reactions. For instance, the individual may think the other person is a bad person (cognition), may feel angered at the other's actions (affect), and their heart rate may increase (arousal). This internal state triggers an automatic appraisal of the situation (e.g., *"this person's behaviour is unforgivable"*). They will then engage in a secondary appraisal, where a deeper consideration of factors such

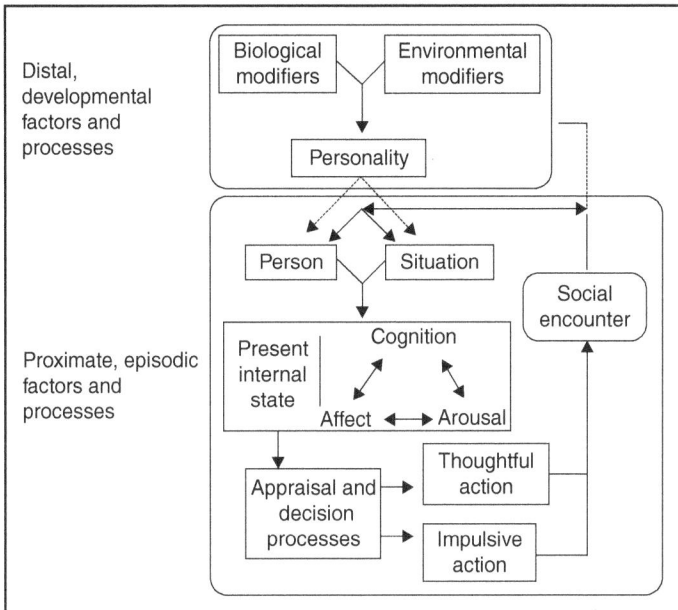

Figure 3.2 Visual representation of the General Aggression Model.

as social rules, the other person's perspective, and anticipated outcomes are considered. The individual's response may then incur a reaction from the other individual(s) which may trigger another interaction, initiating another cycle of appraisal and action.

The feedback loop between social encounters and distal processes represents the constant influence each interaction has on shaping personality. Specifically, the use of aggressive behaviour and appraisal of the outcomes can create aggressive scripts that the individual will then subsequently rely on in similar future situations. The more an individual uses aggression, the more these scripts become readily available and the easier it is for aggressive cognitions to be activated (see Hostile Attribution Bias, discussed below). The integrative nature of GAM allows for an understanding of different forms of violent behaviour and can identify potential strategies for reducing aggression (DeWall & Anderson, 2011; Gilbert et al., 2017).

Cognitive Distortions Associated with Criminality

Cognitive distortions refer to irrational beliefs, attitudes, and thinking patterns that can adversely affect behaviour and wellbeing (Beck, 1963; Ward, 2000). Understanding the distortions held by offenders can help explain how criminal behaviours are rationalised and facilitated. The term 'criminal thinking'

Criminal Thinking. Set of maladaptive thinking patterns and cognitive distortions that enable criminal behaviour.

is used within criminal psychology to denote abnormal attitudes and cognitive distortions commonly held by criminals, which serve to justify and sustain their criminal lifestyles (Walters, 2012).

Walters (1990; also see Walters and White (1989)) developed the Psychological Inventory of Criminal Thinking Styles (PICTS) which identifies eight criminal thinking styles (see Table 3.1) that enable and reinforce criminal engagement and associated deviant behaviour (Walters, 1995, 2006).

Although each thinking style reflects a distinct cognitive bias, most can be categorised as either proactive (promoting planned criminality, 1–4 in Table 3.1) or reactive (impulsive, emotional patterns eliminating internal deterrents, 5–7 in Table 3.1) which facilitate criminal behaviour (Walters, 2006). Whilst most criminal exhibit high levels of criminal thought, they differ in the types of thinking styles styles adopted, with different processes linked to various criminal outcomes. For instance, although all criminal thinking styles are common among prison populations (Walters, 1995), studies show greater endorsement of reactive criminal thinking is associated with substance abuse, future reoffending and an earlier age of initial conviction (Walters, 2020). Thinking styles have also been associated with personalities; reactive criminal thinking commonly associated with emotional disinhibition (e.g., poor impulse control and anger issues), and proactive criminal thinking associated with callous and cruel dispositions (Deblasio & Mojtahedi, 2023). These associations suggest criminal thinking patterns may predict different types of criminal offences, and be informed by personality.

Table 3.1 Criminal Thinking Styles from the Psychological Inventory of Criminal Thinking Styles (PICTS; Walters, 1995).

Criminal thinking style	Description
1. Mollification	Tendency to externalise blame of one's transgressions onto others.
2. Entitlement	Belief that one is entitled to break the law owing to perceived injustices, perceived superiority.
3. Power Orientation	A desire to achieve a sense of power and authority over others.
4. Superoptimism	Inflated beliefs that one can indefinitely avoid negative consequences of criminal behaviour (e.g., arrest).
5. Cognitive Indolence	Over-reliance on taking cognitive short cuts instead of critical reasoning when dealing with problems.
6. Discontinuity	A lack of consistency between an individual's intentions and actual behaviour.
7. Cut-off	Immediately eliminating internal deterrents to offending through substance abuse, mental impairment or short phrases (e.g., "*F*** it!*").
8. Sentimentality	Belief that one is a 'good person' despite their criminal behaviour, often through identification of their other good deeds.

While these criminal thinking styles offer some insight into explaining criminal cognition, they are generalised and do not provide much insight into the thought patterns that inform specific types of offending – which appear to be linked to different cognitive biases (Chereji et al., 2012; Van der Put et al., 2020).

Cognitive distortions associated with violent crime (Hostile Attribution Bias)

An individual is more likely to act aggressively towards another person if they perceive that person to

Hostile Attribution Bias. Inaccurate tendency to interpret the behaviours as having hostile intent.

be hostile. However, assessments of others' intentions are not always accurate. **Hostile Attribution Bias (HAB)** involves the inaccurate tendency to attribute hostile intentions to the behaviour of others – as Dill et al. (1997) aptly put it, people with HAB tend to view the world through blood-red tinted glasses. This Bias can be conceptualised as a cognitive script, shaped through interactions – the more an individual activates the script, the stronger and more accessible it becomes. Individuals possessing a strong HAB are more likely to engage in frequent violent behaviour (Chereji et al., 2012; Yeager et al., 2013). Wegrzyn, Westphal & Kissler (2017) demonstrated this in an experimental study: When presented with images of emotionally ambiguous faces, violent offenders (compared to non-offending participants) were more likely to interpret the faces as being angry.

Cognitive distortions associated with sexual crimes

In the context of sexual offending, cognitive distortions have been criticised for being broad and having incomplete explanations (Ó Ciardha & Ward, 2013). However, there is strong evidence to suggest cognitive distortions can predict risk of sexual offending (Nunes et al., 2016). Ward (2000) referred to these as implicit theories, describing them as deeply ingrained beliefs about the world that serve to justify or rationalise behaviours. Ward framed them as cognitive structures originating from biased cognitive processing, such as erroneous interpretations of social cues. They commonly centre around distorted perceptions of the victims or the self (see Table 3.2), and are frequently endorsed by sex offenders (e.g., Keown et al., 2010; Nunes et al., 2016).

Implicit Theories (of Sexual Offending). Cognitive distortions that serve to support and justify sexual offending.

Neutralisation Theory. Early theory of cognition which identifies thinking styles of criminals which serve to excuse their behaviours.

Victim-focused implicit beliefs portray victim groups as problematic, complicit or unharmed by offender's actions, serving to justify

Table 3.2 Implicit Theories Associated with Sexual Offending.

Implicit Theory	Description
Dangerous World	Belief that the world is a dangerous and hostile place, therefore one must dominate and control others.
Women are problematic	Belief that women are problematic individuals, therefore (sexual) aggression towards them can be justified.
Nature of harm	Belief that sexual molestation is not harmful and is beneficial to children.
Children/Women as sexual beings	Belief that children or women are sexual objects who desire and enjoy sex regardless of consent.
Entitlement	Belief that one is superior to others and as such, entitled to seek out what they desire (in this case, sexual pleasure).
Uncontrollability	Belief that behaviours stemming from one's sexual impulses are out of their control.

sexual violence. The Dangerous World implicit theory corresponds with observations showing that rapists and sexual murderers tend to exhibit more generalised hostility towards others compared to non-offenders (Beech et al., 2005; Vettor et al., 2014). The same implicit theory has also been displayed by some child sex offenders who frame children as being less hostile and dangerous than adults and therefore a more appropriate choice for sexual activity (Ward & Keenan, 1999).

Implicit theories about the offender serve to permit sex offenders to commit their crimes without sanction. Entitlement entails grandiose beliefs that one is entitled to achieve their desires regardless of social or moral rules, reflective of heightened levels of narcissistic traits found in perpetrators of sexual assault (see Mouilso & Calhoun, 2012). The implicit belief of uncontrollability has been observed in child sex offenders, though many rapists of adult women also contend their sexual impulses are uncontrollable (Szumski et al., 2018).

Summary

Understanding the attitudes and cognitive processes behind criminal acts provides valuable insights into explaining, responding to, and preventing crime. While many violent offender interventions lack a theoretical basis (Gilbert & Daffern, 2010), some have highlighted the role cognitive theories of aggression play in rehabilitation (e.g., Fortune & Ward, 2013; Vaske et al., 2011). Beyond violent offending, Andrews and Bonta (2010) identify criminal thinking as a major risk factor for criminal behaviour more generally. However, cognitive models of offending are informative only when understood in conjunction with environmental influences, personality and past experiences.

Further Reading

Journal article – Kersten, R., & Greitemeyer, T. (2024). Human aggression in everyday life: An empirical test of the general aggression model. *British Journal of Social Psychology.* https://doi.org/10.1111/bjso.12718

Video – Short documentary about 'proud paedophile', can you spot any implicit biases/cognitive distortion? (viewer discretion advised): www.youtube.com/watch?v=-XSB4sQGT_4

References

Anderson, C. A., & Bushman, B. J. (2002). Human aggression. *Annual Review of Psychology, 53*(1), 27–51.

Andrews, D. A., & Bonta, J. (2010). Rehabilitating criminal justice policy and practice. *Psychology, Public Policy, and Law, 16*(1), 39.

Bandura, A. (2001). Social cognitive theory: An agentic perspective. *Annual Review of Psychology, 52*(1), 1–26.

Beck, A. T. (1963). Thinking and depression: I. Idiosyncratic content and cognitive distortions. *Archives of General Psychiatry, 9*(4), 324–333.

Beech, A., Fisher, D., & Ward, T. (2005). Sexual Murderers' implicit theories. *Journal of Interpersonal Violence, 21*(11), 166–1389. https://doi.org/10.1177/0886260505278712

Berkowitz, L. (1989). Frustration-aggression hypothesis: Examination and reformulation. *Psychological Bulletin, 106*(1), 59.

Berkowitz, L. (1990). On the formation and regulation of anger and aggression: A cognitive-neoassociationistic analysis. *American Psychologist, 45*(4), 494.

Berkowitz, L. (1993). Affect, aggression, and antisocial behavior. In R. J. Davison, K. R. Scherer, & H. H Goldsmith (Eds.), *Handbook of affective sciences* (p. 815). Oxford University Press.

Berkowitz, L. (2008). On the consideration of automatic as well as controlled psychological processes in aggression. *Aggressive Behavior: Official Journal of the International Society for Research on Aggression, 34*(2), 117–129.

Berkowitz, L. (2012). A cognitive-neoassociation theory of aggression. *Theories of Social Psychology, 2,* 99–117.

Chereji, S. V., Pintea, S., & David, D. (2012). The relationship of anger and cognitive distortions with violence in violent offenders' population: A meta-analytic review. *The European Journal of Psychology Applied to Legal Context, 4*(1), 59.

DeBlasio, S., & Mojtahedi, D. (2023). Exploring the relationship between psychopathy and criminal thinking: Utilising the Tri-PM within a forensic sample. *Journal of Criminological Research, Policy and Practice, 9*(1), 14–30.

DeWall, C. N., & Anderson, C. A. (2011). The general aggression model. In P. R. Shaver & M. Mikulincer (Eds.), *Human aggression and violence: Causes, manifestations, and consequences* (pp. 15–33). American Psychological Association. https://doi.org/10.1037/12346-001

Dill, K. E., Anderson, C. A., Anderson, K. B., & Deuser, W. E. (1997). Effects of aggressive personality on social expectations and social perceptions. *Journal of Research in Personality, 31*(2), 272–292.

Fiske, S. T. (2009). Social cognition. In D. Sander & K. R. Scherer (Eds.), *Oxford companion to emotion and the affective sciences* (pp. 371–373). Oxford University Press.

Fortune, C. A., & Ward, T. (2013). Integrating strength-Based practice with forensic CBT: The good lives model of offender rehabilitation. In R. C. Fortune & D. Mitchell (Eds.), *Forensic CBT: A Handbook for Clinical Practice* (pp. 436–455). Wiley. DOI:10.1002/9781118589878

Gilbert, F., & Daffern, M. (2010). Integrating contemporary aggression theory with violent offender treatment: How thoroughly do interventions target violent behavior? *Aggression and Violent Behavior, 15*(3), 167–180.

Gilbert, F., Daffern, M., & Anderson, C. A. (2017). The General Aggression Model and its application to violent offender assessment and treatment. In P. Sturmey (Ed.), *The Wiley handbook of violence and aggression,* (pp. 1–13). Wiley. DOI: 10.1002/9781119057574

Huesmann, L. R. (1986). Psychological processes promoting the relation between exposure to media violence and aggressive behavior by the viewer. *Journal of Social Issues, 42*(3), 125–139.

Keown, K., Gannon, T. A., & Ward, T. (2010). What's in a measure? A multi-method study of child sexual offenders' beliefs. *Psychology, Crime & Law, 16*(1–2), 125–143.

Mouilso, E. R., & Calhoun, K. S. (2012). Narcissism, psychopathy and five-factor model in sexual assault perpetration. *Personality and Mental Health*, *6*(3), 228–241.

Nunes, K. L., Pettersen, C., Hermann, C. A., Looman, J., & Spape, J. (2016). Does change on the MOLEST and RAPE scales predict sexual recidivism?. *Sexual Abuse*, *28*(5), 427–447.

Ó Ciardha, C., & Ward, T. (2013). Theories of cognitive distortions in sexual offending: What the current research tells us. *Trauma, Violence, & Abuse*, *14*(1), 5–21. https://doi.org/10.1177/152483801 2467856

Szumski, F., Bartels, R. M., Beech, A. R., & Fisher, D. (2018). Distorted cognition related to male sexual offending: The multi-mechanism theory of cognitive distortions (MMT-CD). *Aggression and Violent Behavior*, *39*, 139–151.

van der Put, C. E., Assink, M., & Gubbels, J. (2020). Differences in risk factors for violent, nonviolent, and sexual offending. *Journal of Forensic Psychology Research and Practice*, *20*(4), 341–361.

Vaske, J., Galyean, K., & Cullen, F. T. (2011). Toward a biosocial theory of offender rehabiltiation: Why does cognitive-behavioral therapy work? *Journal of Criminal Justice*, *39*(1), 90–102.

Vettor, S., Beech, A. R., & Woodhams, J. (2014). Rapists and sexual murderers: Combined pathways to offending. In J. Proulx, E. Beauregard, P. Lussier & B. Leclerc (Eds.), *Pathways to sexual aggression* (pp. 285–315). Routledge.

Walters, G. D. (1990). *Criminal lifestyle*. SAGE Publications, Incorporated.

Walters, G. D. (1995). The psychological inventory of criminal thinking styles: Part I: Reliability and preliminary validity. *Criminal Justice and Behavior*, *22*(3), 307–325.

Walters, G. D. (2006). Appraising, researching and conceptualizing criminal thinking: A personal view. *Criminal Behaviour and Mental Health*, *16*(2), 87–99.

Walters, G. D. (2012). Criminal thinking and recidivism: Meta-analytic evidence on the predictive and incremental validity of the Psychological Inventory of Criminal Thinking Styles (PICTS). *Aggression and Violent Behavior*, *17*(3), 272–278.

Walters, G. D. (2020). Predicting future intimate partner violence with past intimate partner violence: The moderating role of proactive and reactive criminal thinking. *Criminal Justice and Behavior*, *47*(8), 943–955.

Walters, G. D., & White, T. W. (1989). The thinking criminal: A cognitive model of lifestyle criminality. *Women Law. J.*, *76*, 4.

Ward, T. (2000). Sexual offenders' cognitive distortions as implicit theories. *Aggression and Violent Behavior*, *5*(5), 491–507.

Ward, T., & Keenan, T. (1999). Child molesters' implicit theories. *Journal of Interpersonal Violence*, *14*(8), 821–838.

Wegrzyn, M., Westphal, S., & Kissler, J. (2017). In your face: the biased judgement of fear-anger expressions in violent offenders. *BMC Psychology*, *5*, 1–12.

Yeager, D. S., Miu, A. S., Powers, J., & Dweck, C. S. (2013). Implicit theories of personality and attributions of hostile intent: A meta-analysis, an experiment, and a longitudinal intervention. *Child Development*, *84*(5), 1651–1667.

Zillmann, D., & Bryant, J. (1974). Effect of residual excitation on the emotional response to provocation and delayed aggressive behavior. *Journal of Personality and Social Psychology*, *30*(6), 782.

Chapter 4

Developmental Theories of Crime

> **Key Points**
>
> Adverse childhood experiences can compromise a child's emotional, cognitive and social development, which can lead to behavioural issues.
>
> Disorganised attachments in infancy can increase the risk of relationship difficulties and criminal behaviour in adult life.
>
> Moffitt's Developmental Taxonomy and the Age-Graded Theory of Informal Social Control explain how adverse childhood experiences can place individuals on a trajectory towards criminal behaviour.

"Villains are not born – they are made"

Renee Bernard in *Lady Falls* (2014)

The quote above is from fiction, but the notion that immoral characters are a product of their environment is a reality that has been evidenced within the fields of psychology and criminology. Developmental theories of crime posit that early adverse childhood experiences can set individuals on a trajectory towards future offending. Childhood is a critical period for cognitive, emotional, and social development (Sartika et al., 2021); consequently, compromised development can lead to emotional and behavioural dysfunction later in life, potentially fostering criminal behaviour (Moffitt, 1993). The case study in Box 4.1. is one of many examples demonstrating

DOI: 10.4324/9781003431213-6

this link. As you read this chapter consider how Aileen's childhood experiences may have shaped her criminal trajectory.

Box 4.1   Case study: Aileen Wuornos.

Aileen Wuornos grew up with little connection to her parents. Her father was never in her life (convicted of child sexual abuse and committed suicide in prison) and her mother abandoned her when she was four. Subsequently, Wuornos lived with her alcoholic grandparents, who subjected her to physical and sexual abuse. By age 11, Wuornos had begun selling her body for drugs, cigarettes and food. At 14, she became pregnant, allegedly after being raped by a family friend, and dropped out of school. At 15, she was ousted from her grandparents' home and began living in the woods, supporting herself through prostitution. In adulthood, Wuornos attempted suicide numerous times and was frequently arrested for various crimes including assault, disorderly conduct, armed robbery and car theft. She would go on to become one of the most infamous female serial killers, robbing and murdering seven men within 12 months.

(Arrigo & Griffin, 2004)

Attachment Theory

According to **Attachment Theory** (Bowlby, 1969), early bonds between an infant and their primary caregiver shape social and emotional development, informing their future interpersonal behaviour. Using the **Strange Situation experiment**, Ainsworth

Attachment Theory. States a child's attachment with their caregiver influences psychological development and future relationships.

Strange Situation Experiment. Experiment where infants are placed in a room with a caregiver who is replaced by a stranger. Thereafter the child is reunited with the caregiver. The child's behaviour is examined at each stage to assess attachment type.

(1979) identified three attachment types, each associated with different patterns of behaviour. Infants with consistently affectionate and attentive caregivers form **secure attachments**, displaying trust towards others. Infants with emotionally distant and unresponsive caregivers form **avoidant attachments**, often exhibiting avoidant or dismissive behaviour towards others. Infants who received inconsistent attention and affection form **anxious/ambivalent attachments**, developing uncertain and insecure attachments to others. A fourth style was proposed by Main and Solomon (1986) –

Secure Attachments. Attachment type characterised by trust, comfort and closeness to others.

Avoidant Attachments. Attachment type characterised by emotional distance and lack of dependency on others.

Anxious/Ambivalent Attachments. Attachment type characterised by fear of abandonment and a strong need for reassurance.

Disorganised Attachment. Attachment type characterised by confusion in relationships resulting in mixed feelings of fear of dependence.

disorganised attachment which describes infants without a clear attachment type who would often freeze or display fear in response to others.

An infant's attachment style is believed to inform the development of **internal working models** – frameworks individuals use to understand the world (Bretherton, 1992). Specifically, insecurely attached infants are more likely

Internal Working Models. Mental framework for perceiving the self and others, developed during childhood.

to develop maladaptive internal working models in relation to affection and attention (Bartholomew & Horowitz, 1991), consequently experiencing greater issues with romantic relationships as adults, particularly in relation to affective communication and intimacy (Loinaz et al., 2021; Muetzelfeld et al., 2020).

Studies have also identified an association between avoidant attachment and sexual coercion (Birnbaum, Weisberg & Simpson, 2011; Davis et al., 2004; Schachner & Shaver, 2004). Karantzas et al. (2016) attributed this to avoidantly attached individuals showing less consideration towards the emotional state of sexual partners, plus a heightened need for control over their partner (Birnbaum et al., 2011). Research also indicates that sex offenders exhibit more disorganised patterns of attachment (Baker et al., 2006; McKillop et al., 2012; Mitchell & Beech, 2011). Grady and Yoder (2024) explained this association by identifying a myriad of interpersonal and behavioural deficits associated with insecure attachment, such as emotional regulation, empathy, aggression and difficulties with intimacy in relationships. Many of these behaviours are common characteristics of **psychopathy**, a personality disorder associated with criminal behaviour which many believe stems from adverse childhood experiences (Schimmenti, 2019; see Chapter 7).

Psychopathy. Personality disorder characterised by antisocial behaviour, lack of empathy and manipulation.

Psychopathy is primarily characterised by affective deficits and behavioural disinhibition, which increase the risk of criminal engagement (McCuish et al., 2021). Psychopaths exhibit significantly more abnormalities in their attachment styles (Schimmenti, 2019), fittingly, many psychopathic traits can be observed amongst insecurely attached children and adults. For instance, studies show that children with avoidant attachments exhibit far less empathy towards the suffering of others (Fowles & Dindo, 2006; Kyranides & Neofytou, 2021; Kyranides et al., 2023) which has been attributed to an impaired ability to regulate negative emotions (Mark et al., 2002). Anxious attachment has been linked to other psychopathic tendencies related to emotional disinhibition (e.g., anxiety and impulsivity), which also makes sense since anxiously attached infants learn to be hostile and suspicious of others (Kyranides & Neofytou, 2021).

While attachment theory helps to illuminate how disrupted childhood attachments may increase the risk of

Desistance. Stopping or reducing criminal activity.

future criminal behaviour, it does not offer a framework for understanding how childhood experiences shape criminal pathways or explain the processes of desistance. The remaining chapter considers two prominent theories surrounding developmental pathways to crime.

Moffitt's Developmental Taxonomy

According to Moffitt's (1993, 2017) **Developmental Taxonomy**, children enter offending through two distinct pathways: **Life-Course Persistent (LCP)** or **Adolescent-Limited (AL)**. Adolescent-Limited offending is primarily caused by social pressure, whereas LCP offending is a product of developmental deficits.

Moffitt's Developmental Taxonomy. Proposes developmental trajectories to crime follow one of two pathways which differ in relation to motivations for offending and desistence.
Life-course Persistent Pathway. Childhood complications render the child more vulnerable to using antisocial behaviour as a coping mechanism throughout life.
Adolescent-limited Pathway. Developmental pathway to delinquency and crime characterised by normative pressures (i.e., peer approval).

Most delinquents follow the AL pathway (Moffitt, 1993). Here antisocial behaviour is driven by normative pressure during adolescence (Chadee, Ali & Burke, 2019), when individuals engage in delinquent behaviours (e.g., substance abuse and minor theft) via association and wanting approval from delinquent peers (Wojciechowski, 2018). This is facilitated by the

maturity gap, (Moffitt, 1993) – a perceived discrepancy between biological and social maturity (including social standing by society). Being denied adult status can lead adolescents to engage in delinquent behaviour to assert their independence.

Maturity Gap. A concept which suggests that adolescents engage in delinquency because their biological maturity outpaces their social maturity and social standing in society.

According to Developmental Taxonomy, the AL pathway eventually leads to desistance when adolescents enter adulthood and take on prosocial roles. Legitimate avenues to social maturity naturally occur (e.g., relationship formation, employment, parenthood) which reduce the maturity gap and shift **reinforcement contingencies** to a point where delinquent behaviour is no longer socially rewarded for

Reinforcement Contingency. Relationship between certain behaviours and their consequences.

them (getting into fights might be considered cool at 12, but not at 30) (Lyon & Welsh, 2017).

Conversely, the LCP pathway presents lifelong antisocial behaviours starting in childhood and persisting into adulthood, becoming more pervasive and leading to serious offending. Causal factors originate from neurological deficits (e.g., hyperactivity, cognitive impairments) and adverse childhood environments (e.g., abuse, neglect, exposure to antisocial behaviour). This interplay can lead children to accept antisocial behaviour as a suitable long term coping mechanism. The same factors can also cause the individual to struggle both socially and academically, impairing their ability to secure employment (Bunting et al., 2018) or form healthy relationships (Pilkington et al., 2021) – both of which are risk factors of offending (Marshall, 2010; Jawadi et al., 2021). As a result, LCP offenders are less likely to possess the resources that enable AL individuals to desist. However, the model can be criticised for being overly deterministic, with little consideration for potential change.

Using a **longitudinal study** following 1,037 male children from the age of three to 26, Moffitt et al. (2002) found as expected, AL

Longitudinal Study. Studies cases over an extended period to identify trends, changes and trajectories.

delinquents demonstrated significantly less antisocial behaviour in adulthood. However, rather than desisting, some of these individuals were still getting into trouble accounting for twice as many property and drug convictions than an unassigned control sample. The researchers argued adulthood may not begin until the age of 25. A study by Wojciechowski (2018) supported this – highlighting desistance may be dependent on individuals dissociating from delinquent peers (which may occur later on).

Age-Graded Theory of Informal Social Control

The **Age-Graded Theory of Informal Social Control** posits that offenders eventually cease offending if subjected to informal social controls – lifestyle factors that indirectly dis-

Age-Graded Theory of Informal Social Control. Theory suggesting the likelihood of engaging and desisting from crime is influenced by life-course transitions and social bonds.

suade such behaviour (Laub et al., 2018; Sampson & Laub, 1993). Examples include attachment to prosocial individuals (e.g., family, peers, or partners) or commitment to prosocial roles which motivate an individual to abstain (e.g., school, employment, or sports).

Sampson and Laub (1993) argue that new informal social controls are encountered at various stages of life through significant life events (**structural turning points**) such as needing employment – which would require moderation of antisocial behaviours to

Structural Turning Point. A significant life event or change that alters an individual's life trajectory, provides new priorities and resultantly influences behaviour (e.g., desistance).

maintain. However, for a structural turning point to exert informal social control, it must be perceived as positive and important by the individual. For instance, if the individual is not satisfied with their job, they are less likely to abstain from offending. The impact will also vary depending on the individual's age – for example someone older may require a higher salary to have their own home or look after a family, and thus may be more motivated to abstain from offending.

Both Moffitt's Developmental Taxonomy and the Age-Graded Theory of Informal Social Control identify prosocial lifestyle changes as important for motivating individuals on criminal trajectories to 'go straight'. This was demonstrated by Peled-Laskov et al. (2019), who found that offenders on parole who were supported in starting a career were less likely to be reincarcerated. However, as both theories elucidate, early developmental risk factors not only promote early delinquency but also reduce desistance opportunities in later life, contributing to offending behaviour continuing. Delinquent children with behavioural disorders may struggle with educational attainment, resulting in further difficulties in employment during adulthood (Bunting et al., 2018; Pilkington et al., 2021). Consequently, these individuals may encounter fewer informal social controls and thus be less inclined to desist. This links to the premise of the Good Lives Model which is discussed in Chapter 15.

Summary

Abnormal childhood experiences can disrupt psychological development potentially leading to antisocial behaviours and criminality. Theories provide insight to understand how pathways to criminality can develop and dissipate. Together, these theories illustrate the interplay of early experiences, social influences and turning points in criminal trajectories.

Further Reading

Journal article – Arrigo, B. A., & Griffin, A. (2004). Serial murder and the case of Aileen Wuornos: Attachment theory, psychopathy, and predatory aggression. *Behavioral Sciences & the Law*, *22*(3), 375–393. https://doi.org/10.1002/bsl.583

Video – Video depiction of Ainsworth's Strange Situation experiment: www.youtube.com/watch?v=QTsewNrHUHU.

Book – Thornberry, T. (Ed.). (2018). *Developmental theories of crime and delinquency.* Routledge.

References

Ainsworth, M. S. (1979). Infant–mother attachment. *American Psychologist, 34*(10), 932.

Arrigo, B. A., & Griffin, A. (2004). Serial murder and the case of Aileen Wuornos: Attachment theory, psychopathy, and predatory aggression. *Behavioral Sciences & the Law, 22*(3), 375–393. https://doi.org/10.1002/bsl.583

Baker, E., Beech, A., & Tyson, M. (2006). Attachment disorganization and its relevance to sexual offending. *Journal of Family Violence, 21*, 221–231. https://doi.org/10.1007/s10896-006-9017-3

Bartholomew, K., & Horowitz, L. M. (1991). Attachment styles among young adults: A test of a four-category model. *Journal of Personality and Social Psychology, 61*(2), 226.

Birnbaum, G. E., Weisberg, Y. J., & Simpson, J. A. (2011). Desire under attack: Attachment orientations and the effects of relationship threat on sexual motivations. *Journal of Social and Personal Relationships, 28*(4), 448–468. https://doi.org/10.1177/0265407510381932

Bowlby, J. (1969). *Attachment and loss* (No. 79). Random House.

Bretherton, I. (1992). Attachment and bonding. In V. B. Hasselt & M. Hersen (Eds.), *Handbook of social development: A lifespan perspective* (pp. 133-155). Springer. https://doi.org/10.1007/978-1-4899-0694-6

Bunting, L., Davidson, G., McCartan, C., Hanratty, J., Bywaters, P., Mason, W., & Steils, N. (2018). The association between child maltreatment and adult poverty–A systematic review of longitudinal research. *Child Abuse & Neglect, 77*, 121–133.

Chadee, D., Ali, S., & Burke, A. (2019). Effects of punishment, social norms, and peer pressure on delinquency: Spare the rod and spoil the child? *Journal of Social and Personal Relationships, 36*(9), 2714–2737.

Davis, D., Shaver, P. R., & Vernon, M. L. (2004). Attachment style and subjective motivations for sex. *Personality and Social Psychology Bulletin, 30*(8), 1076–1090. https://doi.org/10.1177/0146167204264794

Fowles, D. C., & Dindo, L. (2006). A dual-deficit model of psychopathy. *Handbook of Psychopathy, 591*, 14–34.

Grady, M. D., & Yoder, J. (2024). Attachment theory and sexual offending: Making the connection. *Current Psychiatry Reports, 26*(4), 134–141. https://doi.org/10.1007/s11920-024-01488-2

Jawadi, F., Mallick, S. K., Cheffou, A. I., & Augustine, A. (2021). Does higher unemployment lead to greater criminality? Revisiting the debate over the business cycle. *Journal of Economic Behavior & Organization, 182*, 448–471. https://doi.org/10.1016/j.jebo.2019.03.025

Karantzas, G. C., McCabe, M. P., Karantzas, K. M., Pizzirani, B., Campbell, H., & Mullins, E. R. (2016). Attachment style and less severe forms of sexual coercion: A systematic review. *Archives of Sexual Behavior*, *45*, 1053–1068. https://doi.org/10.1007/s10508-015-0600-7

Kyranides, M. N., & Neofytou, L. (2021). Primary and secondary psychopathic traits: The role of attachment and cognitive emotion regulation strategies. *Personality and Individual Differences*, *182*, 111106. https://doi.org/10.1016/j.paid.2021.111106

Kyranides, M. N., Kokkinou, A., Imran, S., & Cetin, M. (2023). Adult attachment and psychopathic traits: Investigating the role of gender, maternal and paternal factors. *Current Psychology*, *42*(6), 4672–4681.

Laub, J. H., Rowan, Z. R., & Sampson, R. J. (2018). The age-graded theory of informal social control. In D. P. Frarington, L. Kazemian & A. R. Piquero (Eds.), *The Oxford handbook of developmental and life-course criminology* (pp. 295–322). https://doi.org/10.1093/oxfor dhb/9780190201371.001.0001

Loinaz, I., Sánchez, L. M., & Vilella, A. (2021). Understanding empathy, self-esteem, and adult attachment in sexual offenders and partner-violent men. *Journal of Interpersonal Violence*, *36*(5–6), 2050–2073. https://doi.org/10.1177/0886260518759977

Lyon, D. R., & Welsh, A. (2017). *The psychology of criminal and violent behaviour*. Oxford University Press.

Main, M., & Solomon, J. (1986). Discovery of an insecure-disorganized/disoriented attachment pattern. In T. B. Brazelton & M. W. Yogman (Eds.), *Affective development in infancy* (pp. 95–124). Ablex Publishing.

Mark, I. L. V. D., IJzendoorn, M. H. V., & Bakermans-Kranenburg, M. J. (2002). Development of empathy in girls during the second year of life: Associations with parenting, attachment, and temperament. *Social Development*, *11*(4), 451–468. https://doi.org/10.1111/1467-9507.00210

Marshall, W. L. (2010). The role of attachments, intimacy, and lonliness in the etiology and maintenance of sexual offending. *Sexual and Relationship Therapy*, *25*(1), 73–85. https://doi.org/10.1080/14681990903550191

McCuish, E., Bouchard, M., & Beauregard, E. (2021). A network-based examination of the longitudinal association between psychopathy and offending versatility. *Journal of Quantitative Criminology*, *37*, 693–714.

McKillop, N., Smallbone, S., Wortley, R., & Andjic, I. (2012). Offenders' attachment and sexual abuse onset: A test of theoretical propositions. *Sexual Abuse*, *24*(6), 591–610. https://doi.org/10.1177/10790632 1244557

Mitchell, I. J., & Beech, A. R. (2011). Towards a neurobiological model of offending. *Clinical Psychology Review*, *31*(5), 872–882. https://doi.org/10.1016/j.cpr.2011.04.001

Moffitt, T. E. (1993) Adolescence-limited and life-course persistent anti-social behaviour: A developmental taxonomy. *Psychological Review*, *100*, 674–701.

Moffitt, T. E. (2017). Adolescence-limited and life-course-persistent anti-social behavior: A developmental taxonomy. In K. M. Beaver (Ed.), *Biosocial Theories of Crime*, (69–96). Routledge. https://doi.org/10.4324/9781315096278

Moffitt, T. E., Caspi, A., Harrington, H., & Milne, B. J. (2002). Males on the life-course-persistent and adolescence-limited antisocial pathways: Follow-up at age 26 years. *Development and Psychopathology*, *14*(1), 179–207.

Muetzelfeld, H., Megale, A., & Friedlander, M. L. (2020). Problematic domains of romantic relationships as a function of attachment insecurity and gender. *Australian and New Zealand Journal of Family Therapy*, *41*(1), 80–90. https://doi.org/10.1002/anzf.1401

Peled-Laskov, R., Shoham, E., & Cojocaru, L. (2019). Work-related intervention programs: Desistance from criminality and occupational integration among released prisoners on parole. *International Journal of Offender Therapy and Comparative Criminology*, *63*(13), 2264–2290.

Pilkington, P. D., Bishop, A., & Younan, R. (2021). Adverse childhood experiences and early maladaptive schemas in adulthood: A systematic review and meta-analysis. *Clinical Psychology & Psychotherapy*, *28*(3), 569–584.

Sampson, R. J., & Laub, J. H. (1993). Crime in the making: Pathways and turning points through life. *Crime & Delinquency*, *39*(3), 396–396. https://doi.org/10.1177/0011128793039003010

Sartika, R., Ismail, D., & Rosida, L. (2021). Factors that affect cognitive and mental emotional development of children: A scoping review. *Journal of Health Technology Assessment in Midwifery*, ISSN, 2620, 5653.

Schachner, D. A., & Shaver, P. R. (2004). Attachment dimensions and sexual motives. *Personal Relationships*, *11*(2), 179–195. https://doi.org/10.1111/j.1475-6811.2004.00077.x

Schimmenti, A. (2019). The developmental roots of psychopathy: An attachment perspective. In S. Itzkowitz & E. Howell (Eds.), *Psychoanalysts, psychologists and psychiatrists discuss psychopathy and human evil* (pp. 219–234). Routledge. https://doi.org/10.4324/9780429262425

Wojciechowski, T. W. (2018). The development of deviant peer association across the life-course and its relevance for predicting offending in early adulthood. *Journal of Developmental and Life-Course Criminology*, *4*, 73–91.

Chapter 5

Social Theories of Crime

Key Points

There are a variety of social and situational theories of crime including:

- labelling theory considering the social construction of crime
- subcultural delinquency and the notion of group identity
- association with criminals
- learning from observation
- the impact of excitement or arousal
- lack of self-control
- relevance of life 'strains'
- routine activity – the presence of a motivated offender, victim and lack of capable guardian

---

Phrases often uttered by parents include 'they got in with the wrong crowd' or 's/he was a bad influence'. Those working in criminal justice may also refer to some having 'no chance' coming from 'that family'. Such muses are also considered by psychologists.

> *Research findings suggest that socialisation processes within families are possibly the largest single source of variation with respect to a child's future risk of involvement in criminal conduct.*
> (McGuire & Duff, 2018, p90)

DOI: 10.4324/9781003431213-7

While this could indicate underlying biological or developmental causation (see Chapters 6 and 4) it also highlights the importance of **social influence** on crime. Things we watch or listen to, people we respect, are friends with or related to, influence our thoughts and behaviour. Children often favour their parent's sports teams, undertake similar careers or follow their attitudes, morals and values. We all remember a family member, friend, teacher, colleague, hairdresser or taxi driver who has guided us at some stage. Other individuals can directly influence our beliefs, decisions and actions.

Social Influence. How people change based on social interactions.

The broader society in which we live can also influence us. A wealthy child, living in a large house, attending private school with access to hobbies and travel has a different life experience to a child living in poverty, caring for a parent, in a run-down flat. As such, wider societal, political, environmental and situational living experiences may also directly influence beliefs, decisions and actions.

Societal influences also include our environment – e.g., inner cities are more likely to suffer high crime than rural areas (e.g., Kokoravec et al., 2021), and crime is more prevalent in narrow, dimly lit alleyways, than in open spaces.

How these **social interactions** and systems (studied by social psychologists), and **situational factors** (explored by criminologists) potentially influence criminal behaviour has been discussed by many disciplines. Some theories are discussed here.

Social Interactions. How people speak or act with one another.
Situational Factors. External influences upon behaviour (as opposed to internal influences such as personality traits).

Labelling

Becker (1963) acknowledged that deviancy is not the act itself, but is socially constructed by the negative labels, rules and sanctions others attach to it. For example, rape in marriage in England and Wales was only included in the Sexual Offences Act in 2003, and gay sex was illegal in India until 2018.

Labelling can be applied to current perceptions of groups like Just Stop Oil – some believing they are legit-

> **Labelling**. Labels are merely social constructs but can become self-fulfilling as people live up to them.

imate environmental campaigners protecting the planet; others thinking their controversial tactics (throwing soup over precious paintings, blocking roads and interrupting events) are criminal (see Further Reading).

Therefore, labelling does not *cause* people to commit crime – but influences whether actions are deemed criminal. However, some argue that someone labelled a criminal, may then self-identify as such, and their offending becomes self-fulfilling. Therefore, rather than regulating behaviour, the stigma of labelling can lead to recidivism. The 'criminal' label may be internalised as part of their identity, and lead to societal rejection. The 'out' group of offenders may form their own 'in' group – enhancing contact with other criminals and increasing their risk of further offending.

Subcultural Delinquency

This notion of revised **social identity** relates to theories of **subcultural delinquency** whereby a new 'subculture' or group identity is formed. McGuire and Duff (2018) highlight that co-offending is the most common form of offending among young people,

> **Social Identity**. How people perceive themselves as part of a group (or not).
> **Subcultural Delinquency**. Delinquent behaviour as a result of group values.
> **Deindividuation**. Losing self-identity when part of a group.

which can lead to **deindividuation** – when those in a crowd may feel reduced accountability for actions. This is reflected in the

Social Identity Model of Deindividuation which states that when people feel anonymous they are more likely to conform to group norms, reducing individual identity and usual moral restraints (Reicher et al., 1995).

> **Social Identity Model of Deindividuation.** Anonymity in a group can lead to heightened conformity to group norms.

Box 5.1   Applications in real life: Gang membership.

Being part of a gang exacerbates personal threats – potentially increasing criminal activity (resulting in a possible criminal record/deprivation of liberties); abuse (e.g., from 'initiations' into a gang); or attracting violence and rivalry (from other gangs).

So why join? Some argue that to achieve a sense of social identity and enhanced self-esteem, a gang can provide cohesion with a group. An 'alternative family' – particularly for those whose actual families are neglectful or not fulfilling basic needs, a gang can provide belonging, garner greater respect, provide elevated status, and establish loyalty from other members.

Levell (2022) reports narratives of gang members outlining the following examples and themes: 'Shaun' highlights the depth of emotional connection *"your feelings for that gang is like mad, it's like love"* (p101), 'Sam' was *"searching for a family, I was searching for love"* (p102) and 'Eric' wanted peer acceptance *"the gang loves you … then you feel accepted"* (p102). The disaffiliation from unmet emotional needs led them to move away from their traditional families, creating new 'gang' connections as an additional, or replacement family.

(see Collier, 1998; Connell, 2005; Levell, 2022)

This is witnessed in gangs as seen in Box 5.1. Underlying problems at home, or in school may lead to association with like-minded peers and internalisation of *their* attitudes, beliefs, values and norms – which may include criminal activity.

Differential Association Theory

Sutherland (1939, 1947) also recognised the importance of others who proposed that criminal behaviour stems from learning via communication and interaction with other criminals. People have **differential or different levels of association** with offenders which determines likely involvement in crime: Those who associate with criminal family members or peers, may learn attitudes and practical methods of how to commit crime. The earlier the contact, the more frequent and longer the interaction, and the closer the association – the greater the likelihood of criminality.

Differential Association. Differing levels of association to criminals can influence participation in crime.

Akers (1973) extended this theory, highlighting how association can be direct – you witness someone committing crime; or indirect – you may have learnt antisocial attitudes from the media. The importance of copying others ('imitation'), and actual or perceived reinforcement – e.g., getting away with the offence and gaining money/kudos from it ('differential reinforcement') were also recognised.

Social Learning Theory/Observational Learning

Bandura et al. (1963) considered *how* people learn via observation. Their experiments demonstrated that children imited aggressive behaviour that they had learnt from adults. More preciesley, children who observed 'model' adults aggresively interacting with a doll (e.g., shouting and hitting the doll) would imitate the aggression when later interacting

Social Learning Theory. How people learn by observing others.

with the doll (children who did not witness aggression did not display aggressive behaviour). Interestingly they did not merely replicate the behaviour but "*invented new ways of attacking the doll*" (Bandura et al., 1963) – for example using guns in addition. Such influence of vicarious learning through an obsession with serial killing is exemplified in Box 5.2.

Box 5.2   Case study: Murder of Brianna Ghey.

On 11 February 2023, 16-year-old Brianna Ghey was stabbed 28 times with a hunting knife in a park in Warrington, UK. A girl and boy (both aged 15) were convicted of murder.

They had exchanged numerous text messages planning the killing and had compiled a list of potential victims. They were preoccupied with violence, torture and death, citing body parts they wished to retain. Notes on serial killers were found in the girl's bedroom and regarding serial killer Richard Ramirez she claimed "*I could talk about him for like two hours, including quotes and dates of stuff*". Her favourite film was Sweeney Todd, which she had watched for "*the 9,000th time*".

www.itv.com/news/granada/2023-11-27/brianna-ghey-boy-and-girl-accused-of-murder-of-transgender-teen-had-kill-list

www.itv.com/news/granada/2023-11-29/shocking-texts-between-murder-accused-teens-read-i-really-want-one-of-its-eyes

---

Perpetration of crime often brings initial reward (e.g., money, excitement) as positive reinforcement – bringing credence to this theory. Moreover, often crime also does not bring punishment as many offences are unreported or offenders remain uncaught.

Excitation Transfer Theory

Social interactions are also considered in **excitation transfer theory**

Excitation Transfer Theory. Heightened arousal from one event can lead to transference to another.

which suggests excitation or arousal from one situation can be carried over into a new context. For example, Zillmann et al. (1972) found transference of prior physical arousal to subsequent aggressive behaviour; and Leclerc and Lindegaard (2018) noted transference of sexual excitation to subsequent sexual offences. This links to the discussion of potential 'triggers' for offences – having an argument at home may lead to arousal, which may be revisited when someone bumps into you later in the day. While usually such an action may be forgiven or perceived as accidental, owing to prior arousal, retention of residual hostility could trigger an aggressive response.

Control Theory

Responsibility for controlling such responses, was considered by Gottfredson and Hirschi (1990) and Hirschi & Gottfredson (1995). They proposed that poor parental teaching of the need for control leads to a later lack of self-control and an inability to resist short-term gains. Individual desires may be met more easily by crime than gain from legitimate means (e.g., stealing something may appear easier than finding and getting a job, working and then saving money to purchase it). Those with little to lose by not conforming to societal rules, or fewer perceived bonds to norms of society, may therefore commit crime.

> **Control Theory**. Bonds to society deter crime. A lack of self-control is associated with crime.

Strain Theories

Strain theories (e.g., Agnew, 1992; Merton, 1938) consider how the want to obtain desirable societal goals (e.g., live in a house) can exert undue pressure or a 'strain' on individuals – particularly when attainment

> **Strain Theory**. How hindrances or an inability to obtain personal goals can lead to strain.

of these goals are hindered via societal influences beyond their control (e.g., they may not be able to gain employment because of inequality in schooling). Offending may occur (e.g., theft) to resolve financial issues (e.g., need money). Strains (such as poverty) can occur when individuals are *prevented* from getting something, but also when *presented* with something or someone negative – for example displaying anger towards an individual who has wronged them (this can be linked to frustration-aggression discussed in Chapter 3).

Routine Activity Theory

Considerations of everyday strains and activities links to Cohen and Felson's (1979) **routine activity theory.** Like everyone, offenders are constrained by available time – they must eat, sleep, etc. As such, unless there is a specific reason to offend in a specified area (for example stealing a specific painting), most offending takes place amidst their everyday, 'routine activity'.

Routine Activity Theory. Crime occurs when an offender and target – without a suitable guardian – come together in time and space.

If a motivated offender comes into contact with a suitable target (person or property) which has inadequate supervision (e.g., a lone female, house without an alarm) in the same time and space – a crime may occur. This is particularly insightful to geographic considerations – people do not have time to travel far, and according to theories of least effort – people are inherently lazy. For example, a perpetrator wanting to steal a mobile phone would not need to travel very far – there would be many suitable targets available nearby. If there is no CCTV or the phone is left unattended (i.e., inadequate supervision) the crime may occur. However, stealing a mobile phone in your own classroom or committing a burglary on your own street provides more limited opportunities (students may have cheaper phones) and may increase the likelihood of being recognised and getting caught. As such offenders display 'buffer zones' or areas which are too risky for them to offend in (e.g., Turner, 1969).

Summary

It seems clear that social and situational factors including association with peers, family, upbringing and living experiences have some role to play in consideration of why some people commit some types of crime (e.g., Maruna, 2021). Juveniles admit that peer influence leads them to engage in crime (Agnew, 1990), and attachment to others can enhance conformity (Hirschi, 2002). Criminal behaviour in groups is therefore likely. We conform to group pressure (e.g., Asch, 1956) and may display obedience even when it involves inflicting suffering on others (e.g., Milgram, 1963). In addition, Brown (2010) highlights that crimes are interpersonal interactions (e.g., between offender and victim) in a 'negotiated transaction' with specific roles and rules. Therefore, the role of social features cannot be overlooked.

Further Reading

Video – Dara was interviewed discussing the offenders responsible for the murder of Brianna Ghey here: www.itv.com/news/granada/2023-12-20/an-experts-take-on-how-two-15-year-olds-became-brianna-gheys-killers

The 2002 documentary 'Bowling for Columbine' by Michael Moore gives a fascinating depiction of the Columbine school massacre in 1999. It highlights some of the theories discussed above, including the potential influence of social learning and environmental influences such as gun laws.

Philip Zimbardo discussed the importance of the social environment in evil acts, considering his infamous Stanford Prison experiment and the parallels to treatment in war here: www.youtube.com/watch?v=5phR pcDyouA#:~:text=Philip%20Zimbado:%20A%20Study%20of,and%20 the%20psychology%20of%20evil.

The interested reader can watch Bandura's experiments into Social Learning Theory here: www.youtube.com/watch?v=NjTxQy_U3ac

Media reports – The current debate in relation to whether groups such as Just Stop Oil are legitimate environmental campaigners or illegal protestors exemplifies labelling theory: www.bbc.co.uk/news/uk-63543307www.bbc.co.uk/news/articles/cly7zy3d3exo

Podcasts – "The Lucifer Effect" how good people can do bad things is discussed on Episode 34 of the podcast "The Psychology of Criminal and Antisocial Behaviour".

References

Agnew, R. (1990). The origins of delinquent events: An examination of offender accounts. *Journal of Research in Crime and Delinquency*, *27*(3), 267–294.

Agnew, R. (1992). Foundation for a general strain theory of crime and delinquency. *Criminology*, *30*(1), 47–88.

Akers, R. L. (1973). *Deviant behavior: A social learning approach.* Wandsworth Publishing Company.

Asch, S. E. (1956). Studies of independence and conformity: I. A minority of one against a unanimous majority. *Psychological Monographs: General and Applied*, *70*(9), 1.

Bandura, A., Ross, D., & Ross, S. A. (1963). Imitation of film-mediated aggressive models. *The Journal of Abnormal and Social Psychology*, *66*(1), 3.

Becker, H. S. (1963). *Outsiders: Studies in the sociology of deviance.* Free Press of Glencoe.

Brown, J. M. (2010). Social psychological theories applied to forensic psychology topics. In J. M. Brown, & E. A. Campbell (Eds.), *The Cambridge handbook of forensic psychology.* Cambridge University Press.

Cohen, L., & Felson, M. (1979). Social change and crime rate trends: A routine activity approach. *American Sociological Review*, *44*, 588–608.

Collier, R. (1998). *Masculinities, crime and criminology.* Sage.

Connell, R. (2005). *Masculinities* (2nd ed.). Routledge. https://doi.org/10.4324/9781003116479

Gottfredson, M. R., & Hirschi, T. (1990). *A general theory of crime.* Stanford University Press.

Hirschi, T. (2002). *Causes of delinquency* (1st ed.). Routledge. https://doi.org/10.4324/9781315081649

Hirschi, T., & Gottfredson, M. R. (1995). Control theory and the life-course perspective. *Studies on Crime & Crime Prevention*, *4*(2), 131–142.

Kokoravec, I., Meško, G., & Marshall, I. H. (2021). Juvenile delinquency and victimisation: Urban vs rural environments. *Revija za kriminalistiko in kriminologijo/Ljubljana*, *72*(4), 323–336.

Leclerc, B., & Lindegaard, M. R. (2018). The emotional experience behind sexually offending in context: Affective states before, during, and after crime events. *Journal of Research in Crime and Delinquency*, *55*(2), 242–277.

Levell, J. (2022). *Boys, childhood domestic abuse, and gang involvement.* Bristol University Press.

Maruna, S. (2021). Criminology, desistance and the psychology of the stranger. In D. Canter & L. Alison (Eds.), *The social psychology of crime* (pp. 287–320). Routledge.

McGuire, J., & Duff, S. (2018). *Forensic psychology: Routes through the system.* Bloomsbury.

Merton, R. (1938). Social structure and anomie. *American Sociological Review, 3*(5), 672–682.

Milgram, S. (1963). Behavioral Study of obedience. *The Journal of Abnormal and Social Psychology, 67*(4), 371–378. https://doi.org/10.1037/h0040525

Reicher, S. D., Spears, R., & Postmes, T. (1995). A social identity model of deindividuation phenomena. *European Review of Social Psychology, 6*(1), 161–198.

Sexual Offences Act 2003, c. 42. www.legislation.gov.uk/ukpga/2003/42

Sutherland, E. H. (1939). *The professional thief.* Chicago University Press.

Sutherland, E. H. (1947). *Principles of criminology* (4th ed.). J. B. Lippincott.

Turner, S. (1969). Delinquency and distance. In T. Sellin & M. E. Wolfgang (Eds.), *Delinquency: Selected studies* (pp. 11–26). John Wiley.

Zillmann, D., Katcher, A. H., & Milavsky, B. (1972). Excitation transfer from physical exercise to subsequent aggressive behavior. *Journal of Experimental Social Psychology, 8*(3), 247–259.

Chapter 6

Neurological Theories of Crime

> **Key Points**
>
> Individuals who suffer traumatic brain injury are more likely to engage in criminality.
> Prefrontal cortex dysfunction can:
>
> - Impair an individual's ability to control impulses (including sexual inhibition)
> - Impair anticipation of consequences of actions
>
> Temporal lobe dysfunction (including amygdala) can:
>
> - Impair ability to recognise and regulate emotions
> - Lead to development of abnormal sexual impulses
>
> Both dysfunctions can increase risk of offending.

Early scientists believed that criminals were neurologically different from non-criminals. Benedikt (1881) believed criminals possessed different brains, identifiable by distinct skull shapes and facial features. Others contended the typical criminal possessed an underdeveloped brain (see Rose & Rose, 2010). Although such beliefs have long been discredited, there is substantial neurological evidence demonstrating a link between brain dysfunction and criminality.

DOI: 10.4324/9781003431213-8

Brain Injury and Criminal Behaviour

Brain dysfunction can arise from numerous genetic and environmental factors, with one of the most common indicators of abnormal brain functioning being traumatic brain injury (**TBI**).

Traumatic Brain Injury (TBI). Brain injury from external force.

While the majority (85–90%) of TBI cases are mild and unlikely to result in permanent damage (Cassidy et al., 2004), severe cases can result in death, physical disability or neurological deficits (NICE, 2014); and multiple (even mild) incidents can lead to significant long-term neurological problems (Wrightson, McGinn & Gronwall, 1995). Traumatic brain inury can result in deficits in cognition (e.g., impulse control, understanding others' perspectives), personality (e.g., aggression, lack of concern), and behaviour (e.g., unemployment, addiction) (Azouvi et al., 2016). Such outcomes can make individuals susceptible to engaging in violent and criminal behaviour (Williams et al., 2018). The prevalence of TBI within the general population is around 8.5% in the US (Silver et al., 2001); within incarcerated populations it can reach 60.2% (Shiroma et al., 2012). Longitudinal studies from Finland (Timonen et al., 2002), Sweden (Fazel et al., 2011) and Australia (Schofield et al., 2015) evidence a clear causal effect of TBI on criminal behaviour. Specifically, individuals with TBI are approximately 1.52–1.6 times more likely to commit crimes than non-injured individuals and 1.65–3 times more likely to commit a violent crime. Such offenders are also more likely to commit crimes at an earlier age and reoffend (Pitman et al., 2015).

Technological advances in brain imaging, such as magnetic resonance imaging (MRI) and functional magnetic resonance imaging (fMRI), have enabled researchers to locate specific regions of the brain, primarily in the **prefrontal cortex (PFC)** and

Prefrontal Cortex (PFC). Frontal region of the brain involved in higher-order cognitive functions (including impulse control, problem-solving and social behaviour).

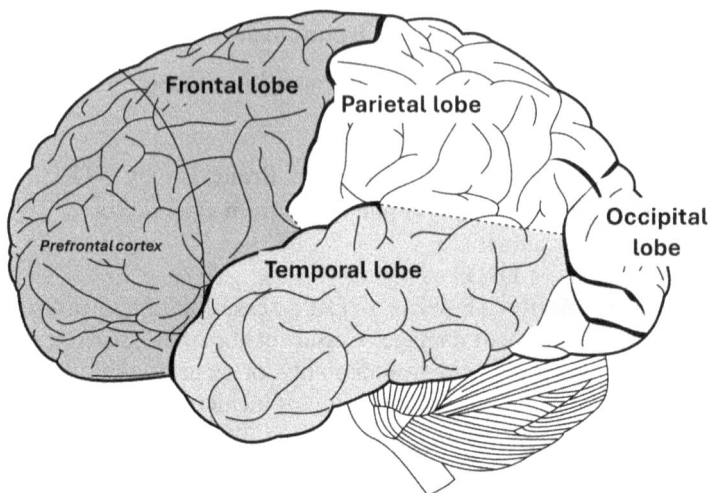

Figure 6.1 Brain regions.

the **temporal lobe**, where dysfunction can increase risk of criminality (see Figure 6.1).

**Temporal Lobe. ** Areas of the brain located behind the ears, responsible for processing and management of senses, emotions, memories and language.

Temporal Lobe Dysfunction

Abnormalities in the temporal lobe, including the **amygdala**, have been linked to aggressive behaviour and offending (Fabian, 2010; Pardini et al., 2014), as well as **Episodic Dysfunction Syndrome** (EDS). This is characterised by frequent outbursts of uncontrollable abnormal behaviours – often violent and unprovoked (Ciesinski et al., 2022).

**Amygdala. ** Small structure within the temporal lobe involved in the processing emotions (particularly fear and pleasure) and formation of emotional memories.

The temporal lobe is responsible for memory encoding, language, processing of visual and auditory information and emotions (Patel et al., 2023). The link between temporal lobe dysfunction and aggression can be attributed to issues with emotional regulation (Davidson et al., 2000). The amygdala processes emotional information from the environment (Dotterer et al., 2020) and when sensing a threat, signals the brain to release stress hormones initiating a fight-or-flight response. Individuals with an overly stimulated amygdala can therefore become more prone to reactive aggression (Blair, 2001). The link between amygdala dysfunction and aggression was further evidenced by Raine et al. (2017) who observed greater levels of amygdala activation in impulsive murderers compared to the general population; additionally other experiments have demonstrated that stimulating the amygdala increases aggression, while inhibiting it electrically (or removing it) reduces agression, rendering the subject docile (Coccaro et al., 2011).

Episodic Dysfunction Syndrome/ Intermittent Explosive Disorder. Condition characterised by frequent outbursts of uncontrollable aggression.

Face-processing (e.g., recognising emotional expressions) is also linked to the amygdala (Anderson et al., 2000) and is important for recognition of fear, distress, and submission from others – markers that can inhibit violent behaviour against them. Specifically, the **violence inhibition mechanism** (VIM) (Blair, 2001) modulates aggression through recognising distress. A damaged or dysfunctional amygdala can create difficulties in recognising anger and fear (Scott et al., 1997). This association between amygdala dysfunction, affect recognition, and criminality is evidenced by criminal psychopaths who display a lack of empathy towards victims (see Chapter 7), deficits in the ability to recognise facial expressions of fear (Hoaken et al., 2007), and reduced amygdala activity during facial processing (Müller et al., 2003).

Violence Inhibition Mechanism. Neurological system that moderates aggression after recognising distress from the recipient.

Temporal dysfunction has also been linked to deviant sexual behaviour (Kaplan & Krueger, 2010). The temporal region is linked to the inhibition of sexual responses, and the surrounding limbic system is involved with pleasure and reward (encompassing sexual arousal) (Unterhorst et al., 2020). Consequently, damage or dysfunction in these regions can result in abnormal and hypersexual behaviour (inability to control sexual impulses) (Jordan et al., 2015).

The **temporal-limbic theory** proposes that damage in temporal and limbic regions can also cause development of abnormal sexual interests such as paedophilia (Dillien et al., 2020). Research found that lesions around the limbic region can cause **hypersexuality** (excessive sexual urges which are difficult to control) and abnormal sexual interests (Spinella et al., 2006). Moreover, neuroimaging techniques identified reduced neuron activity in temporal and limbic regions of child sex offenders compared to controls (Poeppl et al., 2013).

> **Temporal-limbic Theory (of abnormal sexual interest).** Theory suggesting dysfunction within temporal and limbic regions of the brain can cause abnormal sexual interests.
> **Hypersexuality.** Condition involving excessive sexual arousal that is difficult to control.

The link between limbic system damage and sexual deviance was demonstrated in a case involving a woman with long-term multiple sclerosis (MS), an autoimmune disease which causes brain scarring (Ortego et al., 1993). Just before her death, she abruptly developed hypersexuality and various paraphilias, including paedophilia, zoophilia and incest. Inspection of her brain revealed extensive lesions around the limbic (such as the hypothalamus) and temporal regions of her brain.

Prefrontal Cortex Dysfunction

The prefrontal cortex (PFC) plays a significant role in shaping thoughts, behaviours, and personality (Johns, 2014), responsible

for **executive func-
tioning** and emo-
tional regulation.
Executive functions
control behaviour by
monitoring thoughts

Executive Function. Cognitive
skills that help regulate thoughts
and actions to achieve goals.

and selecting or inhibiting behaviours to attain desired goals
(Diamond, 2013). Examples include working memory (temporarily holds information), inhibitory control (to inhibit impulses or
reactions), and cognitive flexibility (adjusting behaviours or shifting focus). Thus, PFC dysfunction can lead to deficiencies in the
ability to plan, control impulses, inhibit inappropriate behaviours,
anticipate consequences, or modify responses (finding alternative, less problematic, solutions) (Blair, 2001). Such deficiencies
can enhance the risk of reacting violently and on impulse. Raine
et al. (1994) observed lower PFC activation during working
memory tasks for violent offenders (compared to non-offenders)
and in a later study (Raine et al., 2017) observed reduced PFC
activity among affective (emotionally provoked) murderers, but
not predatory (planned) murderers. This highlights compromised
behavioural control in reactive violence.

Executive function deficits resulting from abnormal PFC
activity can also increase the risk of sexual offending (Veneziano
et al., 2004). When
presented with sexual
stimuli, paedophilic
offenders show reduced
orbitofrontal cortex
(OFC) and **dorso-
lateral prefrontal
cortex** (DLPFC) acti-
vation (compared
to healthy controls)
(Schiffer et al., 2008),
suggesting dysfunc-

Orbitofrontal Cortex. Region
within PFC involved in emotion,
reward value and reward-related
decision-making.
Dorsolateral Prefrontal Cortex.
Region involved in executive control, emotional processing, and
pain modulation.

tional regions of the brain associated with sexual inhibition. More precisely the OFC has been lined to the inhibition of
sexual arousal and the DLPFC region is involved with inhibitory control, moral reasoning and risky decision-making (Greene

et al., 2004). Szczypiński et al. (2022) used MRI to observe neurological activity of three subject groups (paedophiles who had sexually abused children, paedophiles who had not sexually abused children [demonstrating some inhibition of sexual urges], and healthy non-offending controls) during an experimental game that measured inhibitory control. Findings indicated that paedophilic child abusers possessed weaker inhibitory control and decreased activation in the DLPFC compared to the healthy controls and paedophilic non-child abusers. This suggests while PFC dysfunction may not *cause* paedophilia, the associated inhibition deficits make such groups more inclined to *act* upon abnormal desires. Poeppl et al. (2013) observed similar PFC activation levels between paedophilic child sex offenders and non-paedophilic offenders, reaffirming the link between PFC and child sexual offending results from general inhibitory deficits, rather than an increase in abnormal sexual desire.

Box 6.1 depicts a patient with a tumour purportedly associated with paedophiliac impulses. However, the tumour was in the frontal lobe (linked to sexual *disinhibition* rather than *creation* of abnormal perversion). Resultantly, one might question whether the patient had suppressed paedophilic tendencies prior to the tumour, or whether as claimed, they were caused by the tumour.

Box 6.1   Case study: Tumour associated with paedophilic impulses.

Burns and Swerdlow (2003) describe a case in the United States involving a 40-year-old man with no prior history of paedophilia who suddenly developed an attraction to child pornography. His impulses rapidly escalated, leading him to make sexual advances towards his prepubescent stepdaughter. These were reported, prompting involvement of the authorities. The man was removed from his home and found guilty of child molestation. Prior to sentencing, he sought medical help for a severe headache. He also reported experiencing abnormal thoughts, including suicidal ideation and a fear of raping his landlady. Further abnormal behaviours were observed, such as attempting to solicit nurses for sexual favours and urinating on himself. Doctors discovered a tumour in the right orbitofrontal region of his brain. Removal of the tumour resulted in significant behavioural changes; he no longer exhibited a perversion towards underage children. However, after a year, his headaches and perversion towards child pornography re-emerged. MRI scans later confirmed the tumour had returned to the same region.

Summary

The human brain is a complex structure with many inner workings still not fully understood. It is apparent that brain dysfunction can increase an individual's risk of offending; however, it is not clearly apparent if the relationship between PFC activity and violence is a direct cause. As explored in other chapters, a plethora of inter-related factors may be apparent.

Further Reading

Web article – Natural born killers: brain shape, behaviour and the history of phrenology: https://theconversation.com/natural-born-killers-brain-shape-behaviour-and-the-history-of-phrenology-27518

Video – Documentary on Chris Benoit, a professional wrestler who committed murder and suicide; many believe his actions were a result of sustained brain injuries: www.youtube.com/watch?v=gZklvxk9h2U

Journal Article – Fumagalli, M., Pravettoni, G., & Priori, A. (2015). Pedophilia 30 years after a traumatic brain injury. *Neurological Sciences*, *36*, 481–482. https://doi.org/10.1007/s10072-014-1915-1

References

Anderson, A. K., Spencer, D. D., Fulbright, R. K., & Phelps, E. A. (2000). Contribution of the anteromedial temporal lobes to the evaluation of facial emotion. *Neuropsychology*, *14*(4), 526. https://doi.org/10.1037/0894-4105.14.4.526

Azouvi, P., Vallat-Azouvi, C., Joseph, P. A., Meulemans, T., Bertola, C., Le Gall, D., ... & GREFEX Study Group. (2016). Executive functions deficits after severe traumatic brain injury: The GREFEX study. *The Journal of Head Trauma Rehabilitation*, *31*(3), E10–E20. DOI: 10.1097/HTR.0000000000000169

Benedikt, M. (1881). *Anatomical studies upon brains of criminals*. William Wood & Company.

Blair, R. J. R. (2001). Neurocognitive models of aggression, the antisocial personality disorders, and psychopathy. *Journal of Neurology, Neurosurgery & Psychiatry*, *71*(6), 727–731. https://doi.org/10.1136/jnnp.71.6.727

Burns, J. M., & Swerdlow, R. H. (2003). Right orbitofrontal tumor with pedophilia symptom and constructional apraxia sign. *Archives of Neurology*, *60*(3), 437–440. https://doi.org/10.1001/archneur.60.3.437

Cassidy, D., Carroll, L., Peloso, P., Borg, J., Von Holst, H., Holm, L., ... & Coronado, V. (2004). Incidence, risk factors and prevention of mild traumatic brain injury: Results of the WHO Collaborating Centre Task Force on Mild Traumatic Brain Injury. *Journal of Rehabilitation Medicine*, *30*(43 Suppl.), 28–60.

Ciesinski, N. K., Drabick, D. A., & McCloskey, M. S. (2022). A latent class analysis of intermittent explosive disorder symptoms. *Journal of Affective Disorders*, *302*, 367–375. https://doi.org/10.1016/j.jad.2022.01.099

Coccaro, E. F., Sripada, C. S., Yanowitch, R. N., & Phan, K. L. (2011). Corticolimbic function in impulsive aggressive behavior. *Biological Psychiatry*, *69*(12), 1153–1159. https://doi.org/10.1016/j.biopsych.2011.02.032

Davidson, R. J., Putnam, K. M., & Larson, C. L. (2000). Dysfunction in the neural circuitry of emotion regulation--a possible prelude to violence. *Science*, *289*(5479), 591–594. https://doi.org/10.1126/science.289.5479.591

Diamond, A. (2013). Executive functions. *Annual Review of Psychology*, *64*(1), 135–168. https://doi.org/10.1146/annurev-psych-113011-143750

Dillien, T., Goethals, K., Sabbe, B., & Brazil, I. A. (2020). The neuropsychology of child sexual offending: A systematic review. *Aggression and Violent Behavior*, *54*, 101406. https://doi.org/10.1016/j.avb.2020.101406

Dotterer, H. L., Waller, R., Hein, T. C., Pardon, A., Mitchell, C., Lopez-Duran, N., ... & Hyde, L. W. (2020). Clarifying the link between amygdala functioning during emotion processing and antisocial behaviors versus callous-unemotional traits within a population-based community sample. *Clinical Psychological Science*, *8*(5), 918–935. https://doi.org/10.1177/2167702620922829

Fabian, J. M. (2010). Neuropsychological and neurological correlates in violent and homicidal offenders: A legal and neuroscience perspective. *Aggression and Violent Behavior*, *15*(3), 209–223. https://doi.org/10.1016/j.avb.2009.12.004

Fazel, S., Lichenstein, P., Grann, M., & Langstrom, N. (2011). Risk of violent crime in individuals with epilepsy and traumatic brain injury: A 35-year Swedish population study. *PLOS Medicine.* https://doi.org/10.1371/journal.pmed.1001150

Greene, J. D., Nystrom, L. E., Engell, A. D., Darley, J. M., & Cohen, J. D. (2004). The neural bases of cognitive conflict and control in moral judgment. *Neuron*, *44*(2), 389–400. DOI: 10.1016/j.neuron.2004.09.027

Hoaken, P. N., Allaby, D. B., & Earle, J. (2007). Executive cognitive functioning and the recognition of facial expressions of emotion in incarcerated violent offenders, non-violent offenders, and controls. *Aggressive Behavior: Official Journal of the International Society for Research on Aggression*, *33*(5), 412–421. https://doi.org/10.1002/ab.20194

Johns, P. (2014). *Clinical neuroscience E-book: Clinical neuroscience E-book*. Elsevier Health Sciences.

Jordan, K., Fromberger, P., Müller, J. L., Ralph, N., Rich, P., Turner, D., & Briken, P. (2015). Could we measure sexual interest using functional imaging. *Sexual Offender Treatment*, *10*(1), 1–29.

Kaplan, M. S., & Krueger, R. B. (2010). Diagnosis, assessment, and treatment of hypersexuality. *Journal of Sex Research*, *47*(2–3), 181–198. https://doi.org/10.1080/00224491003592863

Müller, J. L., Sommer, M., Wagner, V., Lange, K., Taschler, H., Röder, C. H., ... & Hajak, G. (2003). Abnormalities in emotion processing within cortical and subcortical regions in criminal psychopaths: Evidence from a functional magnetic resonance imaging study using pictures with emotional content. *Biological Psychiatry*, *54*(2), 152–162. https://doi.org/10.1016/S0006-3223(02)01749-3

NICE. (2014). Head injury: Triage, assessment, investigation and early management of head injury in children, young people and adults. *NICE Clinical Guideline 176.* NICE.

Ortego, N., Miller, B. L., Itabashi, H., & Cummings, J. L. (1993). Altered sexual behavior with multiple sclerosis: A case report. *Cognitive and Behavioral Neurology*, *6*(4), 260–264.

Pardini, D. A., Raine, A., Erickson, K., & Loeber, R. (2014). Lower amygdala volume in men is associated with childhood aggression, early psychopathic traits, and future violence. *Biological Psychiatry*, *75*(1), 73–80. https://doi.org/10.1016/j.biopsych.2013.04.003

Patel, A., Biso, G. M. N. R., & Fowler, J. B. (2023). Neuroanatomy, temporal lobe. StatPearls. https://www.ncbi.nlm.nih.gov/books/NBK519512/

Pitman, I., Haddlesey, C., Ramos, D., Oddy, M., & Fortescue, D. (2015). The association between neuropsychological performance and self-reported traumatic brain injury in a sample of adult male prisoners in the UK. *Neuropsychological Rehabilitation*, *25*(5), 763–779. https://doi.org/10.1080/09602011.2014.973887

Poeppl, T. B., Nitschke, J., Santtila, P., Schecklmann, M., Langguth, B., Greenlee, M. W., ... & Mokros, A. (2013). Association between brain structure and phenotypic characteristics in pedophilia. *Journal of Psychiatric Research*, *47*(5), 678–685. https://doi.org/10.1016/j.jpsychires.2013.01.003

Raine, A., Buchsbaum, M. S., Stanley, J., Lottenberg, S., Abel, L., & Stoddard, J. (1994). Selective reductions in prefrontal glucose metabolism in murderers. *Biological Psychiatry*, *36*(6), 365–373. https://doi.org/10.1016/000-3223(94)91211-4

Raine, A., Meloy, J. R., Bihrle, S., Stoddard, J., LaCasse, L., & Buchsbaum, M. S. (2017). Reduced prefrontal and increased subcortical brain functioning assessed using positron emission tomography in predatory and affective murderers. In K. Beaver (Ed.), *Biosocial theories of crime* (pp. 479–492). Routledge. https://doi.org/10.4324/9781315096278

Rose, H., & Rose, S. (2010). *Alas poor Darwin: Arguments against evolutionary psychology*. Random House.

Schiffer, B., Paul, T., Gizewski, E., Forsting, M., Leygraf, N., Schedlowski, M., & Kruger, T. H. (2008). Functional brain correlates of heterosexual paedophilia. *Neuroimage*, *41*(1), 80–91. https://doi.org/10.1016/j.neuroimage.2008.02.008

Schofield, P., Malacova, E., Preen, D., D'Este, C., Tate, R., Reekie, J., ... & Butler, T. (2015). Does traumatic brain injury lead to criminality? A whole-population retrospective cohort study using linked data. *PLOS One*. *10*(7), e0132558.https://doi.org/10.1371/journal.pone.0132558

Scott, S. K., Young, A. W., Calder, A. J., Hellawell, D. J., Aggleton, J. P., & Johnsons, M. (1997). Impaired auditory recognition of fear and anger following bilateral amygdala lesions. *Nature*, *385*(6613), 254–257. https://doi.org/10.1038/385254a0

Shiroma, E. J., Ferguson, P. L., & Pickelsimer, E. E. (2012). Prevalence of traumatic brain injury in an offender population: A meta-analysis. *The Journal of Head Trauma Rehabilitation*, *27*(3), E1–E10. https://doi.org/10.1097/HTR.0b013e3182571c14

Silver, J., Kramer, R., Greenwald, S., & Wesissman, M. (2001). The association between head injuries and psychiatric disorders: Findings from the New Haven NIMH Epidemiologic Catchment Area Study. *Brain Injury*, *15* (11), 935–945. https://doi.org/10.1080/0269905011 0065295

Spinella, M., White, J., Frank, M. L., & Schiraldi, J. (2006). Neuroanatomical substrates for sex offenses. *International Journal of Forensic Psychology*, *1*(3), 84–94.

Szczypiński, J., Wypych, M., Krasowska, A., Wiśniewski, P., Kopera, M., Suszek, H., ... & Wojnar, M. (2022). Abnormal behavioral and neural responses in the right dorsolateral prefrontal cortex during emotional interference for cognitive control in pedophilic sex offenders. *Journal of Psychiatric Research*, *151*, 131–135. https://doi.org/10.1016/j.jps ychires.2022.04.012

Timonen, M., Miettunen, J., Hakko, H., Zitting, P., Veijola, J., Von Wendt, L., & Räsänen, P. (2002). The association of preceding traumatic brain injury with mental disorders, alcoholism and criminality: The Northern Finland 1966 Birth Cohort Study. *Psychiatry Research*, *113*, 217–226. https://doi.org/10.1016/S0165-1781(02)00269-X

Unterhorst, K., Gerwinn, H., Pohl, A., Kärgel, C., Massau, C., Ristow, I., ... & Ponseti, J. (2020). An exploratory study on the central nervous correlates of sexual excitation and sexual inhibition. *The Journal of Sex Research*, *57*(3), 397–408. https://doi.org/10.1080/00224 499.2018.1539462

Veneziano, C., Veneziano, L., LeGrand, S., & Richards, L. (2004). Neuropsychological executive functions of adolescent sex offenders and nonsex offenders. *Perceptual and Motor Skills*, *98*(2), 661–674. https://doi.org/10.2466/pms.98.2.661-674

Williams, W. H., Chitsabesan, P., Fazel, S., McMillan, T., Hughes, N., Parsonage, M., & Tonks, J. (2018). Traumatic brain injury: A potential cause of violent crime? *The Lancet Psychiatry*, *5*(10), 836–844.

Wrightson, P., McGinn, V., & Gronwall, D. (1995). Mild head injury in pre-school children: Evidence that it can be associated with a persisting cognitive deficit. *Journal of Neurology, Neurosurgery and Psychiatry*, *59*, 375–380

Chapter 7

Clinical Psychological Theories of Crime

Key Points

Mental disorders involving psychosis have been identified as a risk factor for violent crime, though this risk is heavily reduced when factoring out substance abuse.

Personality disorders (PD) are characterised by maladaptive patterns of thinking. Some of these disorders (e.g., narcissist PD and antisocial PD) can promote antisocial and violent behaviour.

Psychopathy, although not a formal clinical diagnosis, is a personality disorder characterised by traits relating to emotional disinhibition and a disregard for the suffering of others. It has been identified as a major risk factor for criminal behaviour.

Occasionally, the media reports criminal acts of extreme cruelty, such as mass murders, which seem inexplicable. This inability to understand underlying motives often leads to assumptions regarding perpetrators being mentally ill and questions about whether such individuals can be treated. This chapter explores the role of mental disorders in violent criminal behaviour. While the list of mental health conditions in clinical diagnosis manuals

Personality Disorders. Condition involving a persistent pattern of maladaptive thoughts, emotions, and behaviours that impair functioning.

DOI: 10.4324/9781003431213-9

are exhaustive, the focus here is on two types of disorders which research has identified as risk factors for crime: conditions involving **psychosis** and **personality disorders.**

Psychosis. Mental state characterised by a loss of contact with reality, typically involving hallucinations, delusions, and impaired thought processes.

Psychosis

Psychosis refers to a collection of symptoms that disconnect an individual from reality, resulting from a combination of genetic (Owen, Craddock & Jablensky., 2007), neurological (Arciniegas et al., 2001), and environmental (Zwicker et al., 2018) factors. Psychosis can occur as a symptom of various mental health conditions. The most notable example is schizophrenia – a chronic mental disorder characterised by hallucinations (typically auditory), delusions, disorganised speech, disorganised behaviour and negative symptoms (e.g., *lack of* emotion or motivation). The **DSM-5-TR** specifies that a diagnosis requires the patient to display at least two of the aforementioned symptoms (of which at least one must be delusions, hallucinations or disorganised speech) for a significant portion of a one-month period (APA, 2022).

Diagnostic and Statistical Manual of Mental Disorders – 5ᵗʰ edition, Text Revision (DSM-5) and International Classification of Diseases (ICD-10). Classifications with diagnostic descriptions of mental health conditions.

Mental health conditions involving psychosis have historically been stigmatised, with many associating them with an increased risk of violence (Wainwright & Mojtahedi, 2020). While it is harmful and inaccurate to label all individuals with major mental health conditions as dangerous, data indicates those with psychotic disorders are overrepresented among violent offenders (Joyal et al., 2007). For example, although only about 0.45% of adults globally have schizophrenia (WHO, 2022), the proportion of homicide offenders with schizophrenia is estimated to be between

5% (Schanda et al., 2004) and 10% (Erb et al., 2001; Wallace et al., 2004). Moreover, Fazel et al. (2009a) found that men with schizophrenia were 4.7 times more likely to commit a violent act than those without the diagnosis.

Command Hallucinations. Auditory third person hallucinations that command the individual to carry out actions.

Schizophrenia. Chronic psychiatric disorder typically characterised by hallucinations, delusions, and disorganised thinking.

Psychosis symptoms such as **command hallucinations** and delusional thought increase the risk of violence (Grohmann et al., 2024). Brucato et al. (2022) reported that 11% of mass murderers had lifetime psychotic symptoms, while Peterson et al. (2024) found that 31% of mass shootings were influenced by psychosis (11% described psychotic symptoms as a major factor). McNiel, Eisner & Binder (2000) found that 30% of psychiatric patients experienced hallucinations commanding them to harm others in the past year, with 22% complying. Patients with such hallucinations were more than twice as likely to be violent, even after accounting for factors like substance abuse. A notable extreme case of supposed psychosis-driven violence is detailed in Box 7.1.

Box 7.1   Case study: Herbert Mullin (Watts et al., n.d.).

Herbert Mullin, had a normal upbringing, with a good academic performance and no evidence of parental abuse (Figure 7.1). However, as he approached adulthood, he struggled with mental health and was diagnosed with paranoid schizophrenia in his mid-twenties. Mullin believed the deaths of Americans during the Vietnam War were blood sacrifices preventing earthquakes in the US, and with the war ending, thought further sacrifices were required. Mullin murdered 13 individuals before being apprehended. Despite his diagnosis, he was tried and convicted owing to evidence of premeditation and attempts to cover his tracks.

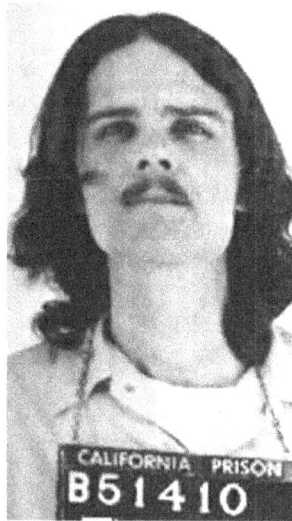

Figure 7.1 Herbert Mullin mugshot.

Large-scale studies indicate that the overrepresentation of those with mental disorders in violent crime diminishes when **comorbidities** and situational factors such as victimisation, economic deprivation, and more notably, substance abuse are accounted for (Elbogen & Johnson, 2009; Swanson et al., 2008). One study found the proportion of psychiatric outpatients who had committed violent offences dropped from 31% to 18% if substance abuse was not present (Monahan et al., 2001). Similar observations were made by Fazel et al. (2009b) when assessing the prevalence of violence among Swedish patients with schizophrenia (27.6% of patients with substance abuse issues; 8.5% without substance abuse issues committed a violent offence). They also compared patients with the

Comorbidity. Simultaneous presence of two or more diseases/health conditions in a patient.

general public, finding individuals with schizophrenia four-to-five times more likely to commit violence. However, when comparing patients with their unaffected siblings (with the same upbringing) they found they were less than twice as likely to commit a violent act, highlighting the importance of genetic and environmental factors. Nevertheless, while confounding factors may inflate associations, robust evidence has demonstrated psychosis still increases the risk of violence, even after controlling for such confounding factors (Hodgins et al., 2003; Swanson et al., 2008).

Personality Disorders

Antisocial personality disorder and narcissistic personality disorder

Personality disorders (PDs) are characterised by long-term patterns of maladaptive thoughts and behaviours. The DSM-5-TR lists 10 PDs, however it is primarily the 'Cluster B' PDs, such as **antisocial personality disorder** (ASPD; also known as Dissocial Personality Disorder in the **ICD-10**) and **narcissistic personality disorder** (NPD), which are frequently observed in offending populations because of their negative impact on emotional behaviour and impulse control (Coid, Moran et al., 2009). Unlike mental disorders characterised by psychosis, 'Cluster B' PDs do not impair an individual's ability to

Antisocial Personality Disorder. Pattern of disregard for the rights of others, characterised by deceitfulness, impulsivity, irritability, aggression, and lack of remorse.

ICD-10. Developed by the World Health Organization, the ICD-10 is a globally used diagnostic tool for diseases and health conditions.

Narcissistic Personality Disorder. Pattern of grandiosity, need for admiration, and lack of empathy, often accompanied by an inflated sense of self-importance.

differentiate right from wrong, meaning such individuals can be deemed fit to stand trial (dependent on other comorbidities).

Narcissistic personality disorder is primarily characterised by a distorted grandiose self-image and intense emotional instability (Tully & Bamford, 2019). Individuals become preoccupied with vanity, power, and superiority, often disregarding others' feelings. Consequently, NPD has been seen as a risk factor for various deviant behaviours including white collar crime, aggressive outbursts, and partner and sexual violence (Russell et al., 2022).

Antisocial personality disorder shares some characteristics but is characterised by irresponsibility, disregard for others' rights and impulsivity and is the strongest PD predictor of violence, with such individuals being between seven to eight times more likely to engage in violent crime and between two to three times more likely to reoffend (Chow et al., 2024).

Evidence suggests both genetic and environmental factors contribute to the development of PDs (Kendler et al., 2019; Rautiainen et al., 2016). Assessments of forensic patients have shown that NPD and ASPD are often linked to adverse childhood experiences involving abuse and/or neglect (Koolen & Keulen-de Vos, 2022). Such experiences can be internalised as **early maladaptive schemas**, influencing behaviours and thoughts in later life (Young et al., 2006). It is therefore common for individuals with these PDs to have other mental health conditions (e.g., substance abuse disorders, Tully & Bamford, 2019).

Early Maladaptive Schemas. Dysfunctional patterns of thinking, often formed through adverse childhood experiences, that continue to distort how individuals perceive themselves, others and the world. This can promote harmful and antisocial behaviour in later life.

Psychopathy

Unlike the PDs mentioned above, psychopathy is not a formal clinical diagnosis listed in the DSM-5. However, the term 'psychopath' is widely recognised as the embodiment of immorality and criminality.

Psychopathy can be understood as a collection of affective, behavioural, and interpersonal characteristics, including a lack of empathy, issues with

Hare Psychopathy Checklist-Revised. Diagnostic tool used to assess psychopathic traits and behaviours.

behavioural control, and a sense of entitlement (Boduszek et al., 2017). As such, some consider psychopathy to be an extreme form of ASPD, however, many of the interpersonal and affective characteristics (described below) are not diagnostic requirements for ASPD.

Psychopathy was originally introduced by Hervey Cleckley (1941) and later operationalised by Robert Hare (1980) into a diagnostic tool which has been refined into what is now considered the gold standard for assessing psychopathy: the Hare Psychopathy Checklist-Revised (PCL-R, Hare, 2003). It consists of 22 items (characteristic, see Table 7.1) scored on a 0 – 2 scale (0 = not present to 2 = definitely present) from clinical interviews and reviews of external sources (e.g., police reports, family statements). A diagnostic cut-off score of 30 is conventionally used to demarcate the presence of psychopathy, although 25 is used in the UK (Skeem et al., 2011).

The individual traits can be problematic, but when presented together significantly increase the risk of violence (Coid et al., 2009). Approximately 1.2% of the general population are considered psychopaths (using the PCL-R, Sanz-García et al., 2021), yet in male prisons, this ranges between 7.7% (Coid et al., 2009) and 25% (Kiehl & Hoffman, 2011). Prisoners with psychopathy show greater pride in their antisocial behaviour (Simourd & Hoge, 2000) and are more likely to reoffend after release (Steadman et al., 2000).

Although the PCL-R is widely endorsed in forensic practice it has faced academic criticism (Evans & Tully, 2016). One is the framework's inclusion of antisocial behaviour as a prerequisite (DeBlasio & Mojtahedi, 2023), even though many psychopaths refrain from breaking the law. 'Corporate psychopaths' work in leadership positions and use charming, manipulative and unempathetic traits to succeed (see Fritzon et al., 2019). Robert Hare

Table 7.1 PCL-R Diagnostic Characteristics.

Factor 1: Interpersonal and Affective Traits		Factor 2: Behavioural/ Lifestyle Traits		Uncategorised Factors
Interpersonal	Affective	Lifestyle	Antisocial	
Glibness/ superficial charm	Lack of remorse or guilt	Prone to boredom	Poor behavioural controls	Promiscuous sexual behaviour
Grandiose sense of self-worth	Shallow affect	Parasitic lifestyle	Early behavioural problems	Many short-term marital relation-ships
Pathological lying	Callous/ lack of empathy	Lack of realistic goals	Juvenile delinquency	
Cunning/ manipula-tive	Failure to accept responsi-bility	Impulsivity	Revocation of conditional release	
		Irresponsi-bility	Criminal versatility	

once remarked, "*If I wasn't studying psychopaths in prison, I'd do it at the stock exchange.*" Another criticism is the PCL-R's categorical assessment approach (you either are or are not a psychopath based on a cut-off score), rather than measuring psychopathy on a continuum (Guay et al., 2007). This led to the conceptualisation of psychopathy as a multidimensional personality construct (e.g., Psychopathic Personality Traits Scale-Revised, Boduszek et al., 2022; Triarchic Psychopathy Measure [Tri-PM], Patrick, 2010). While these self-report scales have limitations (e.g., reduced reliability), they offer a more accessible way to examine psychopathic traits.

Evaluation of Theories of Crime

While certain mental health disorders are associated with an elevated risk of criminal behaviour, this relationship is not deterministic – many individuals with such disorders do not engage in criminal activity. A difficulty with all theories – is that they do not account for all individuals all the time. Psychopaths may do well in corporations. Individuals with law abiding friends, strong role models, and life opportunities may still offend. Some theories may explain some types of crime not others – theft may be motivated by social circumstances (e.g., the need for money) however sexual offences may be linked to personality-based motivations (e.g., the need to control). Imitation from role models may be applicable in burglary or car theft (you get 'taught' by others how to steal), however is less likely in serial homicide (where most offenders act in isolation and have not previously witnessed a murder).

Also, there are methodological difficulties – for example how do you measure concepts such as 'strain'; some theories or assessment tools rely on self-reporting of reasons for behaviours; some experiments are based in the laboratory with limited ecological validity to real world offending; and how do you 'prove' the underlying cause of criminal behaviour by excluding all other variables (such as genes or personality) leaving one genre of features (e.g., cognitive) in explanation alone. In addition, direct causal relationships cannot be determined from correlational studies. It may be for example that rather than being 'led by' peer associates to commit crime (differential association), delinquents may conversely seek out non-law-abiding peers in order to learn.

Summary

We have seen in this chapter how psychosis and personality disorders may link to criminality. However, it is critical to avoid conflating the presence of mental health disorders with a predisposition to criminality, as such assumptions oversimplify the nuanced relationship between mental health and behaviour and contribute to the perpetuation of stigma, which may hinder individuals from accessing treatment. As indicated in the final evaluation section, it is likely that a combination of complex factors cause and perpetuate criminal behaviour.

Further Reading

Journal article – DeLisi, Matt, Alan J. Drury, and Michael J. Elbert. (2019). The etiology of antisocial personality disorder: The differential roles of adverse childhood experiences and childhood psychopathology. *Comprehensive Psychiatry, 92,* 1–6.

Book – Hare, R. D. (1999). *Without conscience: The disturbing world of the psychopaths among us.* Guilford Press.

Podcast – "How Psychopaths Work" by Stuff You Should Know.

References

American Psychiatric Association. (2022). *Diagnostic and statistical manual of mental disorders* (5th ed., text rev.). https://doi.org/10.1176/appi.books.9780890425787

Arciniegas, D. B., Topkoff, J. L., Held, K., & Frey, L. (2001). Psychosis due to neurologic conditions. *Current Treatment Options Neurology, 3,* 347–364. https://doi.org/10.1007/s11940-001-0039-0

Boduszek, D., Debowska, A., McDermott, D., Willmott, D., & Sharratt, K. (2022). Psychopathic Personality Traits Scale–Revised (PPTS-R): Empirical investigation of construct validity and dimensionality in a forensic and non-forensic sample. *Deviant Behavior, 43*(7), 821–828. https://doi.org/10.1080/01639625.2021.1919496

Boduszek, D., Debowska, A., & Willmott, D. (2017). Latent profile analysis of psychopathic traits among homicide, general violent, property, and white-collar offenders. *Journal of Criminal Justice, 51,* 17-23. https://doi.org/10.1016/j.jcrimjus.2017.06.001

Brucato, G., Appelbaum, P. S., Hesson, H., Shea, E. A., Dishy, G., Lee, K., ... & Girgis, R. R. (2022). Psychotic symptoms in mass shootings v. mass murders not involving firearms: Findings from the Columbia mass murder database. *Psychological Medicine, 52*(15), 3422–3430. https://doi.org/10.1017/S0033291721000076

Chow R. T. S., Yu, R., Geddes, J. R., & Fazel, S. (2024). Personality disorders, violence and antisocial behaviour: Updated systematic review and meta-regression analysis. *The British Journal of Psychiatry,* 1–11. https://doi.org/10.1192/bjp.2024.226

Cleckley, H. (1941). *The mask of sanity.* Mosby.

Coid, J., Moran, P., Bebbington, P., Brugha, T., Jenkins, R., Farrell, M., ... & Ullrich, S. (2009). The co-morbidity of personality disorder and clinical syndromes in prisoners. *Criminal Behaviour and Mental Health, 19*(5), 321–333. https://doi.org/10.1002/cbm.747

Coid, J., Yang, M., Ullrich, S., Roberts, A., Moran, P., Bebbington, P., ... & Hare, R. (2009). Psychopathy among prisoners in England and Wales. *International Journal of Law and Psychiatry, 32*(3), 134–141. https://doi.org/10.1016/j.ijlp.2009.02.008

DeBlasio, S., & Mojtahedi, D. (2023). Exploring the relationship between psychopathy and criminal thinking: utilising the Tri-PM within a forensic sample. *Journal of Criminological Research, Policy and Practice*, *9*(1), 14–30. https://doi.org/10.1108/JCRPP-05-2022-0021

Elbogen, E. B., & Johnson, S. C. (2009). The intricate link between violence and mental disorder: Results from the National Epidemiologic Survey on Alcohol and Related Conditions. *Archives of General Psychiatry*, *66*(2), 152–161. https://doi.org/10.1001/archgenpsy chiatry.2008.537

Erb, M., Hodgins, S., Freese, R., Müller-Isberner, R., & Jöckel, D. (2001). Homicide and schizophrenia: Maybe treatment does have a preventive effect. *Criminal Behaviour and Mental Health*, *11*(1), 6–26. https://doi.org/10.1002/cbm.366

Evans, L., & Tully, R. J. (2016). The triarchic psychopathy measure (TriPM): Alternative to the PCL-R? *Aggression and Violent Behavior*, *27*, 79–86. https://doi.org/10.1016/j.avb.2016.03.004

Fazel, S., Gulati, G., Linsell, L., Geddes, J. R., & Grann, M. (2009a). Schizophrenia and violence: Systematic review and meta-analysis. *PLoS Medicine*, *6*(8), e1000120. https://doi.org/10.1371/journal. pmed.1000120

Fazel, S., Långström, N., Hjern, A., Grann, M., & Lichtenstein, P. (2009b). Schizophrenia, substance abuse, and violent crime. *JAMA*, *301*(19), 2016–2023. https://doi.org/10.1001/jama.2009.675

Fritzon, K., Brooks, N., & Croom, S. (2019). *Corporate psychopathy: Investigating destructive personalities in the workplace*. Springer Nature.

Grohmann, M., Kirchebner, J., Lau, S., & Sonnweber, M. (2024). Delusions and delinquencies: A comparison of violent and non-violent offenders with schizophrenia spectrum disorders. *International Journal of Offender Therapy and Comparative Criminology*, 0306624X241248356. https://doi.org/10.1177/0306624X241248356

Guay, J. P., Ruscio, J., Knight, R. A., & Hare, R. D. (2007). A taxometric analysis of the latent structure of psychopathy: Evidence for dimensionality. *Journal of Abnormal Psychology*, *116*(4), 701. https://doi. org/10.1037/0021-843X.116.4.701

Hare, R. D. (1980). A research scale for the assessment of psychopathy in criminal populations. *Personality and Individual Differences*. *1*(2), 111–119. https://doi.org/10.1016/0191-8869(80)90028-8

Hare, R. D. (2003). *Psychopathy checklist—revised. Psychological assessment*. https://doi.org/10.1037/t01167-000

Hodgins, S., Hiscoke, U. L., & Freese, R. (2003). The antecedents of aggressive behavior among men with schizophrenia: A prospective investigation of patients in community treatment. *Behavioral Sciences & the Law*, *21*(4), 523–546. https://doi.org/10.1002/bsl.540

Joyal, C. C., Dubreucq, J. L., Gendron, C., & Millaud, F. (2007). Major mental disorders and violence: A critical update. *Current Psychiatry Reviews*, *3*(1), 33–50. https://doi.org/10.2174/15734000777 9815628

Kendler, K. S., Aggen, S. H., Gillespie, N., Krueger, R. F., Czajkowski, N., Ystrom, E., & Reichborn-Kjennerud, T. (2019). The structure of genetic and environmental influences on normative personality, abnormal personality traits, and personality disorder symptoms. *Psychological Medicine*, *49*(8), 1392–1399. https://doi.org/10.1017/S0033291719000047

Kiehl, K. A., & Hoffman, M. B. (2011). The criminal psychopath: History, neuroscience, treatment, and economics. *Jurimetrics*, *51*, 355.

Koolen, R., & Keulen-de Vos, M. (2022). The relationship between adverse childhood experiences, emotional states and personality disorders in offenders. *Journal of Forensic Psychology Research and Practice*, *22*(1), 18–37. https://doi.org/10.1080/24732850.2021.1945834

McNiel, D. E., Eisner, J. P., & Binder, R. L. (2000). The relationship between command hallucinations and violence. *Psychiatric Services*, *51*(10), 1288–1292. https://doi.org/10.1176/appi.ps.51.10.128

Monahan, J., Steadman, H. J., Silver, E., Appelbaum, P. S., Robbins, P. C., Mulvey, E. P., ... & Banks, S. (2001). *Rethinking risk assessment: The MacArthur study of mental disorder and violence*. Oxford University Press.

Owen, M. J., Craddock, N., & Jablensky, A. (2007). The genetic deconstruction of psychosis. *Schizophrenia Bulletin*, *33*(4), 905–911.

Patrick, C. J. (2010). Operationalizing the triarchic conceptualization of psychopathy: Preliminary description of brief scales for assessment of boldness, meanness, and disinhibition. *Unpublished test manual, Florida State University, Tallahassee, FL*, 1110–1131.

Peterson, J. K., Densley, J. A., Hauf, M., & Moldenhauer, J. (2024). Epidemiology of mass shootings in the United States. *Annual Review of Clinical Psychology*, *20*. https://doi.org/10.1146/annurev-clinpsy-081122-010256

Rautiainen, M. R., Paunio, T., Repo-Tiihonen, E., Virkkunen, M., Ollila, H. M., Sulkava, S., ... & Tiihonen, J. (2016). Genome-wide association study of antisocial personality disorder. *Translational Psychiatry*, *6*(9), e883. https://doi.org/10.1038/tp.2016.155

Russell, T. D., Holdren, S. M., & Ronningstam, E. (2022). Narcissistic personality disorder and deviant behavior. In C. Garofalo & J. J. Sijtsema (Eds), *Clinical forensic psychology: Introductory perspectives on offending*, (pp. 241–268). Springer. https://doi.org/10.1007/978-3-030-80882-2

Sanz-García, A., Gesteira, C., Sanz, J., & García-Vera, M. P. (2021). Prevalence of psychopathy in the general adult population: A systematic review and meta-analysis. *Frontiers in Psychology*, *12*, 661044. https://doi.org/10.3389/fpsyg.2021.661044

Schanda, H., Knecht, G., Schreinzer, D., Stompe, T. H., Ortwein-Swoboda, G., & Waldhoer, T. H. (2004). Homicide and major mental disorders: A 25-year study. *Acta Psychiatrica Scandinavica*, *110*(2), 98–107. https://doi.org/10.1111/j.1600-0047.2004.00305.x

Simourd, D. J., & Hoge, R. D. (2000). Criminal psychopathy: A risk-and-need perspective. *Criminal Justice and Behavior*, *27*(2), 256–272. https://doi.org/10.1177/0093854800027002007

Skeem, J. L., Polaschek, D. L. L., Patrick, C. J., & Lilienfeld, S. O. (2011). Psychopathic personality: Bridging the gap between scientific evidence and public policy. *Psychological Science in the Public Interest*, *12*(3), 95–162. https://doi.org/10.1177/1529100611426706

Steadman, H. J., Silver, E., Monahan, J., Appelbaum, P., Robbins, P. C., Mulvey, E. P., ... & Banks, S. (2000). A classification tree approach to the development of actuarial violence risk assessment tools. *Law and Human Behavior*, *24*, 83–100. https://doi.org/10.1023/A:1005478820425

Swanson, J. W., Swartz, M. S., Van Dorn, R. A., Volavka, J., Monahan, J., Stroup, T. S., ... & Lieberman, J. A. (2008). Comparison of antipsychotic medication effects on reducing violence in people with schizophrenia. *The British Journal of Psychiatry*, *193*(1), 37–43. https://doi.org/10.1192/bjp.bp.107.042630

Tully, R., & Bamford, J. (Eds.). (2019). *Case studies in forensic psychology: Clinical assessment and treatment*. Routledge.

Wainwright, A., & Mojtahedi, D. (2020). An examination of stigmatising attributions about mental illness amongst police custody staff. *International Journal of Law and Psychiatry*, *68*, 101522. https://doi.org/10.1016/j.ijlp.2019.101522

Wallace, C., Mullen, P. E., & Burgess, P. (2004). Criminal offending in schizophrenia over a 25-year period marked by deinstitutionalization and increasing prevalence of comorbid substance use disorders. *American Journal of Psychiatry*, *161*(4), 716–727. https://doi.org/10.1176/appi.ajp.161.4.716

Watts, V., Douglas, V., DeWitt, D., Walker, E., Thompson, K., Stacy, A. V. J., & Soberano, B. (n.d.). Herbert Mullin. Retrieved 14, 2025, from https://maamodt.asp.radford.edu/psyc%20405/serial%20killers/Mullin,%20Herb.pdf

World Health Organization. (2022). Schizophrenia. Retrieved January 14, 2025, from www.who.int/news-room/fact-sheets/detail/schizophre

nia#:~:text=Schizophrenia%20affects%20approximately%2024%20mill
ion,as%20many%20other%20mental%20disorders

Young, J. E., Klosko, J. S., & Weishaar, M. E. (2006). *Schema therapy: A practitioner's guide*. Guilford Press.

Zwicker, A., Denovan-Wright, E. M., & Uher, R. (2018). Gene–environment interplay in the etiology of psychosis. *Psychological Medicine*, *48*(12), 1925–1936.

Part III

Key Methodologies

Chapter 8

Number Crunching (Quantitative Research Methods)

Key Points

Quantitative research methods quantify psychological phenomena for systematic statistical testing.

Quantitative research involves various research designs and methods including experiments, surveys, and secondary data analysis.

Robust methodologies are essential to ensure the findings are reproducible, generalisable and applicable to real-world issues.

Introducing Quantitative Research

Why do psychologists care about statistics so much?

As the coordinator of a university programme on quantitative research methods, I (Dara Mojtahedi) observe two types of psychology students: Those who dislike the topic; and those who do not want to hurt my feelings. I don't blame them as studying quantitative research methods may not be the most appealing aspect of a social science degree, however, such research is crucial for advancing knowledge. Empirical research underpins all scientific disciplines, with teaching, practice, and knowledge stemming from research. Empirical studies employ either quantitative or qualitative approaches (or a combination). While qualitative methods (discussed in Chapter 9) provide rich descriptive

DOI: 10.4324/9781003431213-11

data for exploratory aims and theory development, quantitative research enables us to test and validate these theories as reliable and accurate.

Quantitative research utilises numerical data and statistical methods to systematically investigate psychological phenomena. Behaviours, attitudes, and other characteristics are quantified and analysed statistically to identify patterns, differences, relationships, and causal effects. This approach is essential for testing theories/hypotheses, evaluating interventions, and predicting human behaviour. In forensic and investigative psychology, quantitative research is invaluable for identifying patterns in criminal behaviour, assessing efficacy of prison interventions, testing the reliability of investigative approaches, evaluating legal evidence, and more.

Quantitative methods

Quantitative research can be simplified as studies that explore trends, group differences, or relationships across multiple factors. The methods of exploration vary in complexity. Table 8.1 outlines different quantitative designs and associated research methods. These designs serve various purposes and are not mutually exclusive, with some studies incorporating multiple components.

Experimental research is highly reliable as it allows researchers to manipulate their chosen variable of interest (independent variable) while controlling other variables. Quasi-experimental research offers similar benefits but lacks random allocation to independent variable groups, often using pre-determined groupings (e.g., participant gender). Experimental designs are frequently used in forensic psychology, such as the use of Randomised Control Trials for evaluating forensic interventions (e.g. Shaw et al., 2017), laboratory experiments for testing witness memory (e.g., Mojtahedi et al., 2017) or understanding jury decision-making (e.g. Willmott et al., 2018). However, laboratory-based designs will typically lack **ecological validity** (applicability to real-world situations). David Canter, a pioneer of Investigative Psychology, emphasises the importance of using 'real' data (e.g.,

Ecological Validity. The extent to which a research finding reflects real-world situations.

Table 8.1 Quantitative Methods Used for Data Collection.

Design	Purpose	Key methods	Example
Longitudinal	Studies cases over an extended period to identify trends, changes and trajectories	Cohort studies, panel studies, secondary data analysis	Studying juvenile offenders post-release for up to 15 years, to ascertain whether certain demographic groups are more likely to develop personally disorders (Teplin et al., 2021)
Experiment	Establishes causal relationships by manipulating independent variables and observing the effects on a dependant variable (while controlling for confounding/extraneous variables)	Randomised controlled trials, field experiments, laboratory experiments	Mock juror experiment manipulating the gender and attractiveness of the defendant, and gender of complainant, to see if it effects juror decisions (Winters et al., 2022)
Quasi-experimental	Similar to experimental research without the randomised allocation to independent variable groups	Laboratory experiment, field study	Presenting participants with a sexual exploitation case and measuring their attitudes towards the victim; then testing to see if participants' country of residence and political orientation impacts on victim attitudes (Stevens et al., 2024)

(Continued)

Table 8.1 (Continued)

Design	Purpose	Key methods	Example
Correlational	To examine the relationship between two or more variables without establishing causation	Surveys, observational studies, secondary data analysis	Surveying prisoners to examine whether different psychopathic traits are related to specific criminal thinking biases (DeBlasio & Mojtahedi, 2023)
Descriptive	To identify and describe behaviours, attitudes and characteristics without manipulating variables	Surveys, observational studies, secondary data analysis	Surveying witnesses of serious events to examine the degree to which they discuss incidents with others before and after giving evidence (Paterson & Kemp, 2006)
Meta-analysis	To combine and analyse data from multiple studies to understand trends within the literature	Meta-analysis reviews, secondary data analysis	Reviewing 29 studies to evaluate the pooled effectiveness of psychological interventions in prisons on reducing recidivism (Beaudry et al., 2021)

police data and offender interviews/surveys) to inform practice (Canter & Youngs, 2009).

Longitudinal research can also be experimental or quasi-experimental, considering long-term effects of environmental and genetic factors, making it useful for studying developmental trajectories into crime (Moffitt et al., 2002) and examining long-term intervention effects (e.g. Mann & Reynolds, 2006). However, both longitudinal and experimental designs can be expensive to run.

Descriptive and correlational studies offer less control over variable manipulation and do not allow for causal inferences. However, they are useful for exploratory studies which seek to identify trends and relationships. This includes exploring crime-related attitudes of criminals (e.g., prison studies), laypersons (e.g., attitudes towards victims), and criminal justice professionals (e.g., police officers' perceptions).

Important Considerations

Quantitative research can significantly advance knowledge and has been seen to directly inform criminal justice policy and practice. For example, research on eyewitness identification influenced the use of **double-blind lineup procedures** – reducing the risk of false identification (Wells et al., 2020). However, Riesthuis and Otgaar (2024) highlight that empirical observations *must* be derived from research that is eco-logically valid, replicable, sufficiently sized (dataset) and appropriately interpreted – methodological qualities that are not always present in forensic and investigative psychology research (Nosek et al., 2022; Otgaar et al., 2022).

> **Double-blind Lineup Procedures**. A lineup identification procedure where neither the witness nor the individual administering the lineup is aware which individual in the lineup is the suspect.

Replicability

Quantitative research must be replicable. The ***replication crisis*** reflects concerns about the difficulty of reproducing past research findings, often owing to unclear methods or flaws such as unreliable materials and **p-hacking** (Frias-Navarro et al., 2020). If observations from a study cannot be replicated in subsequent tests, reliability is questionable

Replicability. The ability to replicate the overarching findings of a study by repeating the experiment with new data.

p-hacking. Inappropriate manipulation of data analysis until it produces statistically significant results.

and it remains unknown whether the effect truly exists, or was due to confounding factors. Transparency in methodology and making data available (where permissible) are essential. Research hypotheses should also be grounded in theoretical and/or empirical evidence to reduce the risk of false-positive findings. Using standardised procedures and validated measurements (empirically supported as accurate) can also enhance reliability and comparability. A good example is the Juror Decision Scale (JDS; Willmott et al., 2018), a questionnaire measuring (mock) jurors' appraisals of court cases through three constructs: complainant believability, defendant believability, and verdict confidence. Since development, it has become a popular tool within jury experiments (e.g., Devine & Mojtahedi, 2021).

Effect size interpretation

Most quantitative studies go beyond merely describing the data with frequencies or percentages, using inferential statistics to assess the significance of observed effects or relationships (i.e., evidence that the observation is unlikely to have occurred through chance). **Effect size** is a standardised measure of the magnitude of an observed effect or rela-

Effect Size. A standardised value measuring the strength of a relationship or effect.

tionship. Most can be interpreted according to guidelines (e.g., Cohen, 1988) indicating whether the effect is small, moderate, or large. This standardisation facilitates comparison between studies and helps readers understand real-world implications. Despite its importance, some researchers overlook effect size interpretation, focusing instead on significant p-values (e.g., $p < .05$), providing only partial analysis. A recent review of eyewitness research found that while most studies report effect sizes, few interpreted their meaning (Riesthuis & Otgaar, 2024).

Power analyses

Power analyses are crucial for reliable inferential testing. Researchers must ensure their sample represents the target population, and that the study is sufficiently powered to detect an effect if one exists (avoiding false negatives).

> **Power Analyses.** A measure of the ability of an experimental design and statistical analysis to detect if a particular effect is truly present. Can be used to determine the minimum required sample size for reliably data analysis.

Programmes like G*Power can determine the minimum sample size needed to observe an expected effect size at a specific significance level (e.g., $p < .05$). However, despite power analyses being a standard expectation for reliable quantative analyses, many studies overlook them (Riesthuis & Otgaar, 2024).

Application: Quantitative Research

The studies in Table 8.1 illustrate various quantitative designs within forensic and investigative psychology. Two of these, co-authored by the current author, are detailed below.

Study 1: Examining the relationship between psychopathy and criminal thinking (DeBlasio & Mojtahedi, 2023)

Before academia, Dr Shannon DeBlasio spent almost a decade working in UK prisons, leading on the treatment and rehabilitation of sexual and violent offenders. She encountered a diverse range of prisoners, many presenting psychopathic tendencies; some charming and manipulative, others callous and uninhibited.

DeBlasio noticed a pattern where different psychopathy characteristics appeared to correlate with particular attitudes towards offending. This lead her to consider the relationship between psychopathy and criminal thinking (discussed in Chapter 3) in a research project which I would contribute to.

We employed a correlational design where male inmates from an English prison completed validated questionnaires, including the **Triarchic Psychopathy Measure** (TriPM; Patrick, 2010) and The Psychological Inventory of **Criminal Thinking Styles** (PICTS; Walters, 2001). The TriPM measures three dimensions of psychopathy: disinhibition (e.g., issues with behavioural restraint), meanness (e.g., callousness), and boldness (e.g., fearlessness). PICTS assesses criminal thinking patterns, distinguishing between proactive (cold and collected) and reactive (hot and impulsive) styles.

Triarchic Psychopathy Measure. A self-report questionnaire that measures psychopathy traits.

The Psychological Inventory of Criminal Thinking Styles. A self-report questionnaire that measures different criminal thinking styles.

Meta-analysis Reviews. A review study that combines and analyses the results of multiple studies to draw conclusions about a topic.

Through inferential analysis (regression), we identified clear relationships between psychopathic construct scores and the criminal thinking styles: meanness was the strongest predictor of proactive criminal thinking; disinhibition predicted reactive criminal thinking; and boldness was negatively associated with reactive criminal thinking. This study offered valuable insights, providing practical implications for treatment.

Study 2: Juror decision-making in cases of sexual exploitation (Stevens, Mojtahedi & Austin, 2024)

A research team consisting of the second author and two psychologists from the United States studied the effects of pre-trial attitudes on juror decision-making in sexual exploitation court cases. The study was conceived following research which demonstrated subscription to victim stereotypes and how this impacted on the way victims of sexual violence were treated (e.g., Lilley et al., 2023; Willmott et al., 2024). Similar stereotypes had been observed about victims of sexual exploitation, including from professionals employed to support them (e.g., police officers and medical professionals, see Farrell, 2009; Rajaram & Tidball, 2018). We hypothesised that if such attitudes were endorsed among jurors, victims may be denied justice.

A mock-juror experiment (i.e., simulated court case where participants act as jurors) with a quasi-experimental component was carried out; participants completed a battery of questionnaires measuring demographic characteristics, political ideology and attitudes towards sex trafficking. They then took part in a mock court case involving sexual exploitation, where their verdict, confidence in their decision and perceived believability of both the complainant and defendant, were measured.

Descriptive statistics and regression models were used, identifying that while pre-trial beliefs did not impact on the overall verdict, participants who endorsed inaccurate stereotypical beliefs about victims of sexual exploitation (e.g., it is easy for a victim to escape if they really wanted to) as well as participants who held right-wing beliefs, were more likely to believe the defendant and less likely to believe the complainant.

Summary

While quantitative research may not be the most captivating topic, its importance cannot be overstated. It provides the methodological foundation for testing and validating theories, evaluating interventions, and making predictions. Rigour and reproducibility are paramount, necessitating transparency, theoretical grounding, the use of standardised procedures and validated measures. These considerations ensure the reliability and validity of findings, contributing to the advancement of psychological knowledge and practice.

Further Reading

Book – Field, A. (2024). *Discovering statistics using IBM SPSS statistics*. Sage.
Website – For downloading G*Power:
www.psychologie.hhu.de/arbeitsgruppen/allgemeine-psychologie-und-arbeitspsychologie/gpower.html

Video – Is there a reproducibility crisis in science?
www.youtube.com/watch?v=FpCrY7x5nEE

References

Beaudry, G., Yu, R., Perry, A. E., & Fazel, S. (2021). Effectiveness of psychological interventions in prison to reduce recidivism: A systematic review and meta-analysis of randomised controlled trials. *The Lancet Psychiatry*, *8*(9), 759–773. http://doi. org/10.1016/ S2215-0366(21)00170-X

Canter, D. V., & Youngs, D. (2009). *Investigative psychology: Offender profiling and the analysis of criminal action*. John Wiley.

Cohen, J. (1988). *Statistical power analysis for the behavioral sciences* (2nd ed.). Lawrence Erlbaum Associates.

DeBlasio, S., & Mojtahedi, D. (2023). Exploring the relationship between psychopathy and criminal thinking: Utilising the Tri-PM within a forensic sample. *Journal of Criminological research, Policy and Practice*, *9*(1), 14–30.

Devine, K., & Mojtahedi, D. (2021). Juror decision-making in cases of rape involving high functioning Autistic persons. *International Journal of Law and Psychiatry*, *77*, 101714. https://doi.org/10.1016/ j.ijlp.2021.101714

Farrell, A. (2009). State and local law enforcement responses to human trafficking: Explaining why so few trafficking cases are identified in the United States. In W. F. Mcdonald (Ed.), *Immigration, Crime and Justice* (Vol. *13*, pp. 243–259). Emerald Group Publishing Limited. https://doi.org/10.1108/S1521-6136(2009)0000013016

Frias-Navarro, D., Pascual-Llobell, J., Pascual-Soler, M., Perezgonzalez, J., & Berrios-Riquelme, J. (2020). Replication crisis or an opportunity to improve scientific production?. *European Journal of Education*, *55*(4), 618–631. https://doi.org/10.1111/ejed.12417

Lilley, C., Willmott, D., & Mojtahedi, D. (2023). Juror characteristics on trial: Investigating how psychopathic traits, rape attitudes, victimization experiences, and juror demographics influence decision-making in an intimate partner rape trial. *Frontiers in Psychiatry*, *13*, 1086026.

Mann, E. A., & Reynolds, A. J. (2006). Early intervention and juvenile delinquency prevention: Evidence from the Chicago longitudinal study. *Social Work Research*, *30*(3), 153–167. https://doi.org/10.1093/ swr/30.3.153

Moffitt, T. E., Caspi, A., Harrington, H., & Milne, B. J. (2002). Males on the life-course-persistent and adolescence-limited antisocial pathways: Follow-up at age 26 years. *Development and Psychopathology*, *14*(1), 179–207.

Mojtahedi, D., Ioannou, M., & Hammond, L. (2017). Personality correlates of co-witness suggestibility. *Journal of Forensic Psychology Research and Practice*, *17*(4), 249–27. https://doi.org/10.1080/24732 850.2017.1358996

Nosek, B. A., Hardwicke, T. E., Moshontz, H., Allard, A., Corker, K. S., Dreber, A., & Vazire, S. (2022). Replicability, robustness, and reproducibility in psychological science. *Annual Review of Psychology*, *73*(1), 719–748. https://doi.org/10.1146/annurev-psych-020821-114157

Otgaar, H., Howe, M.L., & Dodier, O. (2022). *What can expert witnesses reliably say about memory in the courtroom? Forensic Science International: Mind and Law*, *3*, 100106. https://doi.org/10.1016/j.fsiml.2022.100106

Paterson, H. M., & Kemp, R. I. (2006). Co-witnesses talk: A survey of eyewitness discussion. *Psychology, Crime & Law*, *12*(2), 181–191. https://doi.org/10.1080/10683160512331316334

Patrick, C.J. (2010). *Operationalizing the triarchic conceptualization of psychopathy: preliminary description of brief scales for assessment of boldness, meanness, and disinhibition*. Florida State University.

Rajaram, S. S., & Tidball, S. (2018). Survivors' voices—Complex needs of sex trafficking survivors in the Midwest. *Behavioral Medicine*, *44*(3), 189–198. https://doi.org/10.1080/08964289.2017.1399101

Riesthuis, P., & Otgaar, H. (2024). An overview of the replicability, generalizability and practical relevance of eyewitness testimony research in the Journal of Criminal Psychology. *Journal of Criminal Psychology*. *15*(2), 176–194. https://doi.org/10.1108/JCP-04-2024-0031

Shaw, J., Conover, S., Herman, D., Jarrett, M., Leese, M., McCrone, P., ... & Stevenson, C. (2017). Critical time Intervention for Severely mentally ill Prisoners (CrISP): A randomised controlled trial. *Health and Social Care Delivery Research*, *5*(8), 1–138. https://doi.org/10.3310/hsdr05080

Stevens, K. L., Mojtahedi, D., & Austin, A. (2024). Juror decision-making within domestic sex trafficking cases: do pre-trial attitudes, gender, culture and right-wing authoritarianism predict believability assessments? *Journal of Criminal Psychology*, *14*(3), 240–258. https://doi.org/10.1108/JCP-09-2023-0059

Teplin, L. A., Potthoff, L. M., Aaby, D. A., Welty, L. J., Dulcan, M. K., & Abram, K. M. (2021). Prevalence, comorbidity, and continuity of psychiatric disorders in a 15-year longitudinal study of youths involved in the juvenile justice system. *JAMA Pediatrics*, *175*(7), e205807.

Walters, G. D. (2001). Revised validity scales for the psychological inventory of criminal thinking styles (PICTS), *Journal of Offender Rehabilitation*, *32*(4),1–13.

Wells, G. L., Kovera, M. B., Douglass, A. B., Brewer, N., Meissner, C. A., & Wixted, J. T. (2020). Policy and procedure recommendations for the collection and preservation of eyewitness identification evidence. *Law and Human Behavior*, *44*(1), 3–36. https://doi.org10.1037/lhb 0000359

Willmott, D., Boduszek, D., Debowska, A., & Woodfield, R. (2018). Introduction and validation of the juror decision scale (JDS): An empirical investigation of the story model. *Journal of Criminal Justice*, *57*, 26–34. https://doi.org/10.1016/j.jcrimjus.2018.03.004

Willmott, D., Rafique, A., Widanaralalage, B. K., & Agneswaran, A. (2024). Investigating the role of psychopathic personality traits, gender and ethnicity in rape myth acceptance. *Psychiatry, Psychology and Law*, 1–13. https://doi.org/10.1080/13218719.2024.2314000

Winters, G. M., Collins, C. M., Kaylor, L. E., & Jeglic, E. L. (2022). The impact of defendant gender and attractiveness on juror decision-making in a sexual offense case. *Deviant Behavior*, *43*(4), 507–524. https://doi.org/10.1080/01639625.2020.1844364

Chapter 9

The Devil is in the Detail (Qualitative Research Methods)

Key Points

Qualitative methods are used to explore research questions.
There are a variety of qualitative methods of data collection (e.g., interviews) and analysis (e.g., thematic analysis).
As opposed to quantitative (numerical) data, qualitative data is textual or visual.
Some studies involve mixed method – incorporating qualitative and quantitative.

Qualitative Methods

Qualitative methods are used to explore **research questions** in depth. For example, we may enquire why people commit crime by interviewing offenders – obtaining a holistic picture of their life and circumstances. While quantitative methods rely upon standardised, objective collection of measurable numerical or categorical data; **qualitative data** can

Research Questions. Questions a study seeks to answer (compared to hypotheses which are testable predictions about relationships between variables).

Qualitative Data. Non-numerical information e.g., speech, text.

DOI: 10.4324/9781003431213-12

involve speech, interviews, focus groups or any text – including on-line comments or chat. In a questionnaire enquiring about victimisation, quantitative questions may ask victims to 'tick boxes' regarding the type or number of offences they have experienced. Qualitative questions may have **'free text' options** in which respondents are asked to write how they felt about these experiences and what are the long-term effects. Thus, qualitative analysis often seeks to understand the underlying *meaning* for those involved.

Free Text Options. Respondents write their own answer in their own words.

Examples of some qualitative methods of data collection and how they have been used in forensic and investigative psychology are outlined in Table 9.1.

Both the method of data collection, and the type of analysis required, depends upon the research question

Ethnographic Study. Researchers immerse themselves to observe and collect data on a particular culture or community.

trying to be answered. Examples of some of those used in the research outlined in the final column of Table 9.1 are described in Table 9.2. These are not exhaustive but merely identify some common types – there are many methods of data collection and analysis available (see further reading) and each provides explicit guidelines to the researcher on how to appropriately conduct the research.

Application: Qualitative Research

The first author has recently been involved in two predominantly qualitative research projects considering domestic violence and abuse (DVA). Both used a combination of surveys, interviews and focus groups with **participants** including the public, victims/survi-

Participants. Individuals who actively participate in research, providing data – e.g., interviewees.

vors, perpetrators, and professionals working in the field. Parts of

Table 9.1 Qualitative Methods Used for Data Collection.

Method	Of use for	Example
Interview	In depth analysis of individual experiences. Can be structured, semi-structured, or unstructured	Interviewing offenders about their experiences attending youth offending support (King et al., 2014)
Focus group	Focussed discussion of topics instigated by the researcher, by a small group	Discussing with prisoners and staff how a prison environment influences mental health (Nurse et al., 2003)
Use of secondary data	Use of pre-existing data not primarily collected for the purposes of research – e.g., witness statements	Analysing published speeches of those promoting hate crime (Rasaq et al., 2017)
Case study	Detailed study of a certain individual, organisation, group or entity	Analysing documents regarding a police officer who abused his position for sexual purpose (Sweeting & Cole, 2022)
Observation	Watching a situation or events without attempting to manipulate or change it	Ethnographic study involving observation of a murder investigation team (Innes, 2003)
Survey	Ascertaining the views of many individuals in writing	A survey to explore accessibility to domestic violence and abuse diversion programmes (Harvey et al., 2024)

these studies are considered to highlight the reasons for different methods of data collection, the analysis and brief findings.

Study 1: Exploration of perpetrator support programmes (Levell et al., 2021)

The first study involved a European research collaboration between five countries (Cyprus, Greece, Italy, Romania and the UK) exploring perpetrator support programmes for those

Table 9.2 Qualitative Methods of Data Analysis.

Method	Of use for
Thematic Analysis (Braun & Clarke, 2022)	Identification of underlying patterns (themes) within data
Interpretive Phenomenological Analysis (Smith et al., 1999)	Eliciting how individuals make meaning of their life experiences
Grounded Theory (Glaser & Strauss, 2017)	Exploration of data without any prior preconceptions or ideas when there is little or no previous knowledge on the topic
Discourse Analysis (Potter & Wetherell, 1987)	Analysis of language or discourse, considers nuances such as pauses and emphasis in speech

engaged in domestic violence and abuse (DVA). The aim was to elicit best practice and make recommendations for future programmes (Levell et al., 2021). One part involved interviews with 18 individuals who had previously perpetrated domestic violence and abuse and were receiving support from services. We wanted to explore how they experienced accessing of support, and what they found useful (or otherwise).

Why interviews?

Interviews were chosen for several reasons. First, they are private – taking place with only one or two interviewers. They can be in person, on the phone or on-line (e.g., via the Zoom/Teams programs). As such the participants need not be seen and can maintain anonymity – particularly appropriate for dealing with sensitive topics that people might be reluctant to discuss in a group (Milena et al., 2008). In addition, the interviews were semi-structured – there were suggested questions, but if the individual brought up something of interest to the research, this could be probed and explored. The interviewer therefore had more scope to investigate points made by the participant, and go off on raised 'tangents', if relevant. Thus, compared to a survey or structured interview, the research is more personalised and may gain deeper insights than merely answering fixed questions.

There can however be barriers to conducting interviews. Gaining access to participants can be difficult – you may not know where to find them and many may not want to take part or not turn up. Moreover, there are considerable ethical challenges – for example contingencies need to be considered regarding what to do if the perpetrator discloses criminal activity or indicates someone may be in danger. If face to face the physical safety of the researchers needs to be ensured. In addition, the content of the interview cannot be predicted, and the researcher may have to listen to disturbing information or harrowing disclosures which may negatively affect them. Such risks need to be considered in advance. Practically there may also be barriers – where should interviews take place for privacy and to minimise interruption, and what happens if there are Wifi connection issues or recordings of transcripts fail. Also, interviews can be lengthy – some participants talk continuously, others struggle for words. As such conducting interviews (or focus groups) can be difficult, requiring significant pre-planning, practise, advice and support.

Box 9.1   Applications in real life: Eliciting data.

Although any interview is likely to have a schedule of questions, estimated times and potential prompts (e.g., who, what, where, why, how, when), it is usual to experience instances where both participants do not stop talking; and where interviewees have little to say. Both can be difficult to negotiate. Unlike chairing a meeting of focussed agenda items, curtailing a senior police officer talking about a high-profile case they have worked on may lessen valuable data collection; or cutting off a survivor telling their narrative of abuse can be rude and potentially immoral, if not unethical. Conversely if participants have little to say, getting information can be difficult. Prompts can elicit interaction; however, in focus groups some participants say far more than others. Specific prompts can assist in opening the floor to engagement from others including: 'What does anyone else think?'; 'Do any of you disagree or agree with this?' If people have agreed to participate it is likely they will, yet if they have

> little to say this cannot be forced. This should be carefully considered in focus groups in particular – for example if senior and junior or less experienced staff are in the same group, depending on the personalities of the individuals and dynamics of the organisation, some staff may feel less confident in contributing. In such instances running different groups or alternative interviews/surveys may be worthwhile.

This is exemplified in Box 9.1.

What was asked?
In our study, participants were asked to describe their experiences of obtaining support for changing their abusive behaviour, and how they thought services could be improved. Questions were developed to answer the research questions in conjunction with support service specialists, cognisant of the overall aim of the funded research. They were asked about the ease or otherwise of accessing support and its availability; what interventions worked for them; and how they felt it impacted on their subsequent behaviour.

What was done?
The interviews with perpetrators were undertaken and transcribed, and a step-by-step method of thematic analysis (see Braun & Clarke, 2022) was conducted looking for repeated patterns within the data which were summarised into codes. Similar codes were then grouped into overall, identified themes to consider the research questions.

Themes. Overarching ideas or patterns that emerge from qualitative data.

What was found?
Despite being from different countries, there was consistency between participants, in that many described significant barriers to engaging with services – 'barriers' was one of the identified themes. For example, an initial barrier was some participants

did not acknowledge their behaviour was wrong. Particularly when violence was not physical, the consequences of emotional or controlling behaviour were not initially recognised. Others highlighted that calling an initiative a 'perpetrator' programme brought negative associations and put individuals off engaging owing to embarrassment, guilt and shame. Comments included,

> *People think I'm a bad man. (Bogdan)*
> *It's a horrible, horrible title. (Bob)*

Other barriers were also noted – a lack of funding or awareness of perpetrator programmes, or difficulties in accessing them,

> *I did not go because it was during work. (Bogdan)*
> *I drive 65 kilometres each time to go to the programme. (Vasil)*

The full report (Levell et al, 2021) details other findings, but this section highlights how from interviews and understanding the experiences and perspectives of the perpetrators, deeper meaning was explored subsequently leading to suggestions for practice.

Study 2: Minority groups access to domestic abuse services (Cole et al., 2025)

The second study involved collaboration with two charities who wanted to explore services for victims/survivors of domestic abuse from Black and Ethnic Minority (BME), Lesbian Gay Bisexual Transgender Queer Intersex and Asexual (LGBTQIA+) and disabled communities (Cole et al., 2025). The overall aim was to consider current service provision, identify bespoke requirements of these groups, and make recommendations to improve practice. The study involved focus groups, interviews and surveys of the general public (including those from all communities; and those who had or had not experienced or received support for DVA). We only discuss the survey here.

A total of 317 people responded which included both tick box and free text responses. This highlights that

Mixed Method. Researchers collect both quantitative (numerical) and qualitative (descriptive) data.

this research was a **mixed method** design – i.e., involving both quantitative and qualitative data. While we focus on the qualitative elements, you will observe that some percentages of **respondents** are cited reflecting the quantitative elements and the usefulness of this integration.

Respondents. Those who respond providing data – e.g., individuals who complete surveys.

Why survey?

Surveys were chosen to obtain views from a broad section of society within a geographic area. An on-line survey was disseminated via social media, and via 88 charities, community groups and other organisations/institutions, for example those specialising in support for BME, LGBTQIA+ and disabled people. Incorporating 'free text' boxes allowed respondents to articulate their own views. In addition, the surveys were private, anonymous and could be completed at any time, in any place convenient.

There were initial difficulties in obtaining respondents, so perseverance was required to publicise it more widely. Ethical considerations included that respondents: had to give consent for their data to be used, were informed in advance of the nature of the survey, were made aware that they did not have to answer every question, were informed how the findings would be used, understood their right to withdraw their responses (how to do so/the time to do so), and that respondents knew where they could find further support or information regarding subsequent findings.

What was asked?

Respondents were asked about services accessed (if any), what worked well, what could be improved, and support needs (both in general, and in relation to the specific communities of focus).

What was done?

From the free text responses, thematic analysis (Braun & Clarke, 2022) was conducted. A **coding 'template'** was compiled,

Coding Template. Structured framework to label data.

which drew on existing knowledge and other parts of the study. An example code was 'having a voice' when someone mentioned they or others needed to be heard or listened to. Codes were then grouped into overall themes – for example 'having a voice' was merged with other codes such as 'length of time' (consideration of the length of time things took) into the overall theme of 'needs' which reflected the needs of victims/survivors when seeking assistance from support services.

What was found?
Nearly 70% of respondents had previously used support services for DVA, including many from the targeted communities, with over half saying the services received were useful or very useful. One respondent stated (under the theme of 'good practice')

> *Without their support I would not have been able to leave and I would likely not be alive.*
>
> (Fleur)

A further theme considered 'general needs' by all victim/survivors. From quantitative tick boxes the services that respondents felt were most needed, included access to mental health and counselling support, however from the qualitative free text boxes it was clear some needs were not being met.

> *I wasn't given counselling until my physical health was sorted. (Cathy)*
> *Opportunities to be able to meet with other women with similar experiences. (Josie)*

Needs of specific groups were also recognised under a separate theme of 'bespoke needs.'

> *Language barriers and cultural differences may mean people are unable to access services. (Ruby)*
> *Those with disabilities may find it difficult to leave an abuser. (Alice)*
> *The main thing I think would help is autism friendly shelter. (Ella)*

Such findings therefore provided an evidence base for the need for funding of bespoke services for victims/survivors from certain groups.

Summary

There are a variety of research methods and types of qualitative analysis. The method used is dependent on the research question trying to be answered. Two examples of qualitative research alongside ethical considerations have been explored highlighting how a more detailed understanding of meaning and issues pertinent to respondents can be gleaned from in depth, qualitative consideration.

Further Reading

Book – There are many books detailing the different methods of data collection and analysis available to researchers including Lyons, E., & Coyle, A. (Eds.). (2021). *Analysing qualitative data in psychology*. Sage.

Websites – Details of the first study described above (Levell et al., 2021) can be found at www.osspc.eu/app/

The second study (Cole et al., 2025) has also been published here www.mdpi.com/2076-328X/15/2/103

Videos – Victoria Clarke on YouTube (@victoriaclarke592) provides a series of videos on Thematic Analysis.

Podcasts – The podcast "BP Psychology" simply explores qualitative methods, Episode 86 specifically discusses 'Quantitative vs Qualitative Data', Episode 86 looks at 'observations', and Episode 79 explores the importance and detriments of 'case studies'.

References

Braun, V., & Clarke, V. (2022). *Thematic analysis: A practical guide*. Sage.

Cole, T., Harvey, O., Healy, J., & Smith, C. (2025). Contemporary treatment of crime victims/survivors: Barriers faced by minority groups in accessing and utilizing domestic abuse services. *Behavioral Sciences, 15*(2), 103.

Glaser, B., & Strauss, A. (2017). *Discovery of grounded theory: Strategies for qualitative research*. Routledge.

Harvey, O., Cole, T., Levell, J., & Healy, J. (2024). Explorations of attitudes towards accessibility and accessing domestic violence and abuse

(DVA) perpetrator support programmes by victim-survivors and per-petrators across five European countries. *Abuse: An International Impact Journal, 5*(1), 26–45.

Innes, M. (2003). *Investigating murder.* Oxford University Press.

King, E., Brown, D., Petch, V., & Wright, A. (2014). Perceptions of support-seeking in young people attending a Youth Offending Team: An interpretative phenomenological analysis. *Clinical Child Psychology and Psychiatry, 19*(1), 7–23.

Levell, J., Healy, J., Cole, T., Harvey, O., & Pritchard, C. (2021). The other side of the story: Perpetrators in change. *Time for Change.* Retrieved Jan 25, 2025 from www.osspc.eu/app/sites/default/files/inline-files/2021_OSSPC_Time_for_Change_Report.pdf

Milena, Z. R., Dainora, G., & Alin, S. (2008). Qualitative research methods: A comparison between focus-group and in-depth interview. *Annals of the University of Oradea, Economic Science Series, 17*(4), 1279–1283.

Nurse, J., Woodcock, P., & Ormsby, J. (2003). Influence of environ-mental factors on mental health within prisons: Focus group study. *British Medical Journal, 327*(7413), 480.

Potter, J., & Wetherell, M. (1987). *Discourse and social psychology.* Sage.

Rasaq, A., Udende, P., Ibrahim, A., & Oba, L. A. (2017). Media, politics, and hate speech: A critical discourse analysis. *E-Academia Journal, 6*(1), 240–252.

Smith, J. A., Jarman, M., & Osborn, M. (1999). Doing interpretative phenomenological analysis. *Qualitative Health Psychology: Theories and Methods, 1*(1), 218–240.

Sweeting, F., & Cole, T. (2022). *PC "Just-do-enough"–A retrospective case study of a police officer who abused his position for a sexual purpose.* Unpublished eprint. Retrieved March 10, 2025 from https://eprints.bournemouth.ac.uk/37460/

Part IV

Key Impacts

Chapter 10

Eyewitness Evidence

Key Points

Eyewitnesses play a significant role in investigations, helping direct inquiries, identifying suspects, and providing evidence in court. However, inaccuracies can mislead investigations and contribute to false convictions.

Eyewitness research has identified a range of factors that can influence the accuracy of memory reports including stress/arousal, presence of a weapon, and post-event information.

Contradictions in eyewitness research have been primarily the result of methodological differences in the way memory has been measured, with some laboratory experiments lacking ecological validity.

Importance of Witness Reports

Eyewitnesses play a crucial role in many criminal investigations, often providing pivotal information that can shape investigative strategies and influence legal proceedings (Otgaar & Howe, 2018). Witnesses can assist law enforcement by explaining how an incident unfolded, as well as describing and identifying persons of interest. However, when errors are made, consequences can be significant. A review of 375 wrongful convictions for serious crimes revealed 69% of cases involved inaccurate eyewitness

DOI: 10.4324/9781003431213-14

testimony (Innocence Project, 2024). The case of Stephen Titus (Box 10.1) exemplifies this. Wrongful convictions can incur long lasting detrimental effects for those wrongfully convicted (see Brooks & Greenberg, 2021), law enforcement (reputationally and financially, Lipscombe & Beard, 2015) and the community (as the real perpetrators are free to reoffend).

Box 10.1   Case study: Taken from The Seattle Times (Henderson, 1981).

On October 12, 1980, a female hitchhiker was raped in Washington, US. The victim described the assailant as being 25–30 years old, having a beard, and wearing a three-piece suit. She described his vehicle as royal blue with cloth seats and recalled seeing a large brown folder inside.

Later that day, officers pulled over Stephen Titus (Figure 10.1, left) as he was driving home with his partner. Titus had a beard and drove a royal blue car, although he was not wearing a suit, and his car did not have cloth seats. Officers also claimed to have found a large brown folder in the vehicle, but Titus argued the folder had been planted after his arrest.

Initially, the victim picked Titus out of a lineup, saying he looked *most* like the offender. At the trial, she reaffirmed her belief, stating Titus was *definitely* the attacker. Titus was convicted of first-degree rape but fortunately, the charges were dismissed later that year when the real perpetrator, a serial rapist named Edward Lee King (Figure 10.1, right). was charged with the offence. However, the consequences were significant: Titus struggled with long-term unemployment, significant financial loss, and the end of his relationship with his partner (Figure 10.1).

Research has informed investigative and legal professionals on factors that can impair the accuracy of eyewitness memory and suspect identification. The current chapter reviews three factors that have been at the at the centre of academic debate.

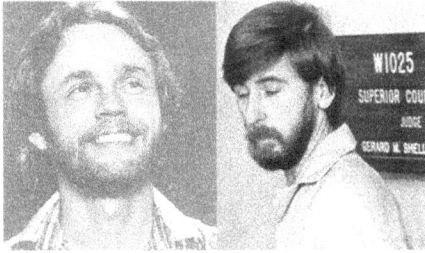

Figure 10.1 Images of Stephen Titus [left] and Edward Lee King [right].

Detriments of Memory Report Accuracy

Stress and anxiety

Encountering a criminal incident can trigger acute stress and arousal within the witness which can negatively affect their ability to accurately recall information (Loftus, 1979). Pezdek et al. (2021) tested the effects of stress on memory recall in an experiment that presented participants with images that were either stress-inducing or non-stress inducing. When participants were later asked to identify the faces from the images, the authors noticed a drop in facial recognition accuracy for faces from the stress-inducing images. Shortcomings of the study included stress levels not being directly measured, and exposure to an image not evoking a similar level of stress as witnessing a crime. Valentine and Mesout (2009) overcame these limitations in a field experiment, where visitors of an immersive horror attraction had their stress and anxiety levels measured and were later asked to describe the performer. Participants who displayed higher levels of stress and anxiety provided fewer correct descriptors, more incorrect details, and were more likely to make false identifications from a lineup, compared to those with lower levels.

In contradiction however, some have failed to find a relationship between stress and memory accuracy (e.g. Christianson & Hübinette, 1993; Sauerland et al., 2016), and some studies evidence that stress at the encoding stage of memory can actually improve later recall (see Shields et al., 2017). There is academic disagreement, with 78% of human memory researchers believing that experiencing stress during an event enhances memory, but only 32% of those specialising in *eyewitness* memory share this belief (Marr et al., 2021). Marr et al. (2021) suggest the contradictory findings result from differences in choice of stressors, measurements used, and the intervals between observation and retrieval. Nevertheless, when focusing on studies involving high levels of stress, there is overwhelming evidence demonstrating a clear negative effect on recall and identification (see Deffenbacher et al., 2004).

The weapon focus effect

Stress during a criminal incident can be heightened if a weapon is brandished. In particular, the presence of a gun can significantly reduce accuracy of witness statements (Davies et al., 2008; Steblay, 1992). An early **weapon focus effect** study by Loftus, Loftus and Messo (1987) presented participants with a series of slides depicting an interaction

Weapon Focus Effect. Inhibiting effect on memory accuracy resulting from exposure to a weapon.

between a cashier and a customer. Participants viewed images of a customer either brandishing a gun or presenting a cheque. The authors found more time was spent fixating on the gun than on the cheque, and participants in the first ("gun") condition demonstrated poorer memory for the incident. The effect has been replicated (e.g. Hope & Wright, 2007; Pickel, 2009), though more recent developments suggest the weapon will only reduce memory if fully brandished (not if concealed – Carlson et al., 2017). The visual presence of a weapon, rather than just knowledge of its presence, appears necessary for it to impact later recall.

Arousal/Threat Hypothesis. Suggests the threatening nature of a weapon induces physiological arousal which inhibits memory.

There are competing theoretical explanations for why a weapon inhibits memory. The **arousal/ threat hypothesis**

(Kramer et al., 1990) posits that a weapon's threatening nature induces physiological arousal, causing individuals to fixate on the source of stress (Easterbrook, 1959). While this is plausible, most experiments have presented the weapon through videos, which evoke far less physiological arousal. Furthermore, research does not find the weapon focus effect when the weapon is consistent with the context (e.g., seeing a police officer carry a gun, Pickel et al., 2008).

An alternative explanation is the **unusual item hypothesis.** This suggests that items considered incongruous with activated schemas (expectations based

Unusual Item Hypothesis. Suggests an item considered to be incongruent with its environment will demand visual attention.

on previous knowledge) capture attention owing to requiring further interpretation (Loftus & Mackworth, 1978). Thus, a witness encountering a weapon during an incident will become fixated on the item as it deviates from their typical expectations. However, in cases where the weapon may be expected (such as seeing police officers holding a gun), the weapon is not considered incongruent therefore, it does not draw the viewer's focus (Pickel et al., 2008). The unusual item hypothesis was supported by Hope and Wright (2007), who found other incongruent items, such as a celery stick, have the same inhibiting effect as a weapon on memory. The case study outlined in Box 10.2 demonstrates the absurd nature of the offence which drew witnesses' attention, limiting awareness of the perpetrator's appearance. However, Hope and Wright (2007) compared the effects of both an unusual item and a weapon against a control condition and found that while both the unusual item and the weapon led to poorer memory recall compared to a control condition, participants who viewed a weapon also exhibited poorer recall for peripheral items compared to participants who viewed the unusual item. This suggests that both the unusualness and the stress-inducing nature of a weapon may affect memory consolidation and future recall.

Box 10.2   Case study: Robbery (Fawcett et al., 2013).

In 1997, a robber entered a coffee shop in Toronto, Canada and threatened to kill a hostage unless the bystanders handed over money. The terrified onlookers complied with his demands and paid him to leave the hostage unharmed. What makes this case unusual is that the robber did not brandish a weapon, nor did he take a hostage from within the coffee shop. The hostage was a Canada Goose the robber brought with him into the store, threatening to kill it if his demands were not met. The unusual nature of this incident caused witnesses to focus their attention on the poor, frightened goose rather than the robber's appearance, which consequently affected their ability to recall the perpetrator's appearance later on.

Further complications in understanding the true effects of weapons arise when considering **archival research**. Studies that have analysed witness testimonies from past cases have failed to demonstrate a weapon

Archival Research. Uses data from real cases (e.g., legal reports) rather than from experiments.

focus effect (Behrman & Davey, 2001). Horry et al. (2014) failed to find a relationship between weapon presence and suspect identification; contrary to laboratory studies, the authors did find that weapon-present crimes were slightly less likely to result in foil-identification (i.e., the witness identifying the wrong person from a lineup), compared to weapon-absent crimes.

Post-event information

After witnessing an incident, eyewitnesses may encounter new 'post-event' information about the incident

Post-event Information. Information about a witnessed event learnt from an external source.

from external sources such as the media, other witnesses or investigators (Gabbert et al., 2012). Although interviewers typically encourage witnesses to recall only what they personally observed, studies suggest eyewitnesses are susceptible to including misleading post-event information in their statements, a phenomenon know as the **misinformation effect** (Loftus, 2005).

Misinformation Effect. When misleading post-event information contaminates a witness's recollection of the event.

Laboratory experiments have demonstrated that participants encountering post-event information about a witnessed incident have then recalled this (incorrect) information in subsequent reports (Carlucci et al., 2010; Mojtahedi et al., 2018). This includes the false reporting of person/suspect characteristics (Mojtahedi et al., 2025; Nourkova Bernstein & Loftus, 2004), as well as key details about the event, including the blaming of innocent bystanders for the offence (Mojtahedi et al., 2017; Mojtahedi et al., 2019).

Witnesses can incorporate misleading post-event information into their memory intentionally or unintentionally. Intentional misinformation acceptance is the result of **informational influence**, whereby an individual chooses to conform to external sources even if it contradicts their own judgements owing to perceiving the external source to be correct

Informational Influence. Where an individual chooses to conform to external sources even if it contradicts their own judgements owing to perceiving the external source as correct.

(Wright et al., 2009). This conformity has been evidenced by studies showing misinformation acceptance rates differ depending on the perceived confidence (Goodwin et al., 2012) and credibility of the source (Mojtahedi et al., 2020). Unintentional

Source Monitoring Errors. Misattribution of the source from which a memory was learnt.

misinformation acceptance can occur following **source monitoring errors** – whereby the source of the post-event information is mistakenly assumed to come from the incident (i.e., witnessed) and thus, included during memory reconstruction (Landau & Marsh, 1997).

While an overwhelming body of evidence leaves no doubt about the effects of misinformation on recall, much evidence is from experiments that purposely presented participants with believable misinformation. It is unclear how frequently co-witnesses encounter inaccurate information during discussions in reality, or whether such information is contested. Moreover, recent field research by van Rosmalen and Vredeveldt (2025) suggests collaborative interviewing (interviewing witnesses together) may be beneficial for individual recall. The authors observed real police interviews where witnesses were interviewed individually and later alongside co-witnesses (where they may have encountered new information). Witnesses were able to recall additional details from the incident when collaborating with a co-witness, suggesting that without artificial inclusion of misinformation, co-witness discussion could enhance recall accuracy.

Summary

This chapter examined factors that can lead to inaccurate recollections. There are many case examples demonstrating the detriments of unreliable memory – the misallocation of police resources from the false identification of a second suspect in the Oklahoma Bomber investigation (see Wright, Self & Justice, 2000) and the wrongful conviction of Barry George (Gabbert & Hope, 2013) to name a few. While it is crucial to understand the conditions under which eyewitness testimony can be unreliable, it is also important to acknowledge potential publication bias in the literature, which often focuses on eyewitness errors. Human memory is a powerful tool and plays a vital role in solving many criminal investigations, but research into understanding these errors is needed to ensure witness evidence is used reliably.

Further Reading

Video – TED talk by Elizabeth Loftus on the reliability of memory: www.youtube.com/watch?v=PB2OegI6wvI

Journal article – Case study of the Oklahoma bombing which demonstrates the misinformation effect: Memon, A., & Wright, D. B. (1999). Eyewitness testimony and the Oklahoma bombing. *The Psychologist.*
Podcast – "How Eyewitness Testimony Works (?)" by *Stuff You Should Know*

References

Behrman, B. W., & Davey, S. L. (2001). Eyewitness identification in actual criminal cases: An archival analysis. *Law and Human Behavior*, *25*(5), 475–491. https://doi.org/10.1023/A:1012840831846

Brooks, S. K., & Greenberg, N. (2021). Psychological impact of being wrongfully accused of criminal offences: A systematic literature review. *Medicine, Science and the Law*, *61*(1), 44–54. https://doi.org/ 10.1177/0025802420949069

Carlson, C. A., Dias, J. L., Weatherford, D. R., & Carlson, M. A. (2017). An investigation of the weapon focus effect and the confidence–accuracy relationship for eyewitness identification. *Journal of Applied Research in Memory and Cognition*, *6*(1), 82. https://doi.org/ 10.1037/h0101806

Carlucci, M., Kieckhaefer, J., Schwartz, S., Villalba, D., & Wright, D. (2010). The South Beach study: Bystanders' memories are more malleable. *Applied Cognitive Psychology*, *25*(4), 562–566. http://dx.doi. org/10.1002/acp.1720

Christianson, S. Å., & Hübinette, B. (1993). Hands up! A study of witnesses' emotional reactions and memories associated with bank robberies. *Applied Cognitive Psychology*, *7*(5), 365–379. https://doi.org/ 10.1002/acp.2350070502

Davies, G. M., Smith, S., & Blincoe, C. (2008). A "weapon focus" effect in children. *Psychology, Crime & Law*, *14*(1), 19–28. https://doi.org/ 10.1080/10683160701340593

Deffenbacher, K., Bornstein, B., Penrod, S., & McGorty, E. (2004). A meta-analytic review of the effects of high stress on eyewitness memory. *Law and Human Behavior*, *28*(6), 687–706. http://dx.doi.org/ 10.1007/s10979-004-0565-x

Fawcett, J. M., Russell, E. J., Peace, K. A., & Christie, J. (2013). Of guns and geese: A meta-analytic review of the 'weapon focus' literature. *Psychology, Crime & Law*, *19*(1), 35–66. https://doi.org/10.1080/ 1068316X.2011.599325

Gabbert, F., & Hope, L. (2013). Suggestibility and memory conformity. In A. M. Ridley, F. Gabbert & D. J. La Rooy (Eds.), *Suggestibility in legal contexts: Psychological research and forensic implications* (pp. 63–83). Wiley. DOI:10.1002/9781118432907

Gabbert, F., Hope, L., Fisher, R., & Jamieson, K. (2012). Protecting against misleading post-event information with a self-administered interview. *Applied Cognitive Psychology*, 26(4), 568–575. http://dx.doi.org/10.1002/acp.2828

Goodwin, K., Kukucka, J., & Hawks, I. (2012). Co-witness confidence, conformity, and eyewitness memory: An examination of normative and informational social influences. *Applied Cognitive Psychology*, 27(1), 91–100. http://dx.doi.org/10.1002/acp.2877

Henderson, P. (1981). Looking back at Titus case. *The Seattle Times*. July 2, 1981. https://special.seattletimes.com/o/news/local/tituscase/lookingback.html

Hope, L., & Wright, D. (2007). Beyond unusual? Examining the role of attention in the weapon focus effect. *Applied Cognitive Psychology: The Official Journal of the Society for Applied Research in Memory and Cognition*, 21(7), 951–961. https://doi.org/10.1002/acp.1307

Horry, R., Halford, P., Brewer, N., Milne, R., & Bull, R. (2014). Archival analyses of eyewitness identification test outcomes: What can they tell us about eyewitness memory? *Law and Human Behavior*, 38(1), 94.

Innocence Project. (2024). *DNA exonerations in the United States*. www.innocenceproject.org/dna-exonerations-in-the-united-states/

Kramer, T. H., Buckhout, R., & Eugenio, P. (1990). Weapon focus, arousal, and eyewitness memory: Attention must be paid. *Law and Human Behavior*, 14(2), 167. http://dx.doi.org/10.1007/BF01062971.

Landau, J., & Marsh, R. (1997). Monitoring source in an unconscious plagiarism paradigm. *Psychonomic Bulletin & Review*, 4(2), 265–270. http://dx.doi.org/10.3758/bf03209404

Lipscombe, S., & Beard, J. (2015) Research briefing: Miscarriages of justice: compensation schemes. *House of Commons Library*. https://commonslibrary.parliament.uk/research-briefings/sn02131/

Loftus, E. F. (1979). The malleability of human memory: Information introduced after we view an incident can transform memory. *American Scientist*, 67(3), 312–320.

Loftus, E. F. (2005). Planting misinformation in the human mind: A 30-year investigation of the malleability of memory. *Learning & Memory*, 12(4), 361–366. http://dx.doi.org/10.1101/lm.94705

Loftus, E. F., Loftus, G. R., & Messo, J. (1987). Some facts about "weapon focus". *Law and Human Behavior*, 11(1), 55–62. https://doi.org/10.1007/BF01044839

Loftus, G. R., & Mackworth, N. H. (1978). Cognitive determinants of fixation location during picture viewing. *Journal of Experimental Psychology: Human Perception and Performance*, 4(4), 565. https://doi.org/10.1037/0096-1523.4.4.565

Marr, C., Sauerland, M., Otgaar, H., Quaedflieg, C. W., & Hope, L. (2021). The effects of acute stress on eyewitness memory: An integrative review for eyewitness researchers. *Memory*, *29*(8), 1091–1100. https://doi.org/10.1080/09658211.2021.1955935

Mojtahedi, D., Ioannou, M., & Hammond, L. (2017). Personality correlates of co-witness suggestibility. *Journal of Forensic Psychology Research and Practice*, *17*(4), 249–27. https://doi.org/10.1080/24732 850.2017.1358996

Mojtahedi, D., Ioannou, M., & Hammond, L. (2018). Group size, misinformation and unanimity influences on co-witness judgments. *Journal of Forensic Psychiatry & Psychology*, *29*(5), 844–865. https://doi.org/ 10.1080/14789949.2018.1439990

Mojtahedi, D., Ioannou, M., & Hammond, L. (2020) Intelligence, authority, and blame conformity: Co-witness influence is moderated by the perceived competence of the Information Source. *Journal of Police and Criminal Psychology*, 1–10. https://doi.org/10.1007/s11 896-019-09361-2

Mojtahedi, D., Ioannou, M., Hammond, L., & Synnott, J. P. (2019) Investigating the effects of age and gender on co-witness suggestibility during blame attribution. *Journal of Investigative Psychology and Offender Profiling*, *16*(3), 153–168. https://doi.org/10.1002/ jip.1533

Mojtahedi, D., Williams, T., Hunt, D., Ioannou, M., Synnott, J., Tzani, C., & van der Kemp, J. J. (2025). Can metamemory judgements predict the risk of memory contamination for facial descriptions? *Legal and Criminological Psychology*. https://doi.org/10.1111/ lcrp.12313

Nourkova, V., Bernstein, D., & Loftus, E. (2004). Altering traumatic memory. *Cognition and Emotion*, *18*(4), 575–585. https://doi.org/ 10.1080/02699930341000455

Otgaar, H., & Howe, M. L. (2018). When children's testimonies are used as evidence: how children's accounts may impact child custodial decisions. *Journal of Child Custody*, *15*(4), 263–267.

Pezdek, K., Abed, E., & Cormia, A. (2021). Elevated stress impairs the accuracy of eyewitness memory but not the confidence–accuracy relationship. *Journal of Experimental Psychology: Applied*, *27*(1), 158–169. https://doi.org/10.1037/xap0000316

Pickel, K. L. (2009). The weapon focus effect on memory for female versus male perpetrators. *Memory*, *17*(6), 664–678. https://doi.org/ 10.1080/09658210903029412

Pickel, K. L., Narter, D. B., Jameson, M. M., & Lenhardt, T. T. (2008). The weapon focus effect in child eyewitnesses. *Psychology, Crime & Law*, *14*(1), 61–72. https://doi.org/10.1080/09658210903029412

Sauerland, M., Raymaekers, L. H., Otgaar, H., Memon, A., Waltjen, T. T., Nivo, M., ... & Smeets, T. (2016). Stress, stress-induced cortisol responses, and eyewitness identification performance. *Behavioral Sciences & the Law*, *34*(4), 580–594. https://doi.org/10.1002/bsl.2249

Shields, G. S., Sazma, M. A., McCullough, A. M., & Yonelinas, A. P. (2017). The effects of acute stress on episodic memory: A meta-analysis and integrative review. *Psychological Bulletin*, *143*(6), 636. https://doi.org/10.1037/bul0000100

Steblay, N. (1992). A meta-analytic review of the weapon focus effect. *Law and Human Behavior*, *16*(4), 413–424. http://dx.doi.org/10.1007/bf02352267

Valentine, T., & Mesout, J. (2009). Eyewitness identification under stress in the London Dungeon. *Applied Cognitive Psychology: The Official Journal of the Society for Applied Research in Memory and Cognition*, *23*(2), 151–161. https://doi.org/10.1002/acp.1463

van Rosmalen, E. A., & Vredeveldt, A. (2025). Collaborative interviewing of eyewitnesses: A field study. *Journal of Criminal Psychology*, *15*(2), 210–226. http://dx.doi.org/10.1108/JCP-04-2024-0028

Wright, D., London, K., & Waechter, M. (2009). Social anxiety moderates memory conformity in adolescents. *Applied Cognitive Psychology*, *24*(7), 1034–1045. http://dx.doi.org/10.1002/acp.1604

Wright, D., Self, G., & Justice, C. (2000). Memory conformity: Exploring misinformation effects when presented by another person. *British Journal of Psychology*, *91*(2), 189–202. http://dx.doi.org/10.1348/000712600161781

Chapter 11

Behavioural Analysis of Crime

<hr>

> **Key Points**
>
> Behavioural Analysis is not just about offender profiling but can provide a range of assistance to investigations.
>
> There are a variety of roles including Crime Analysts, Behavioural Investigative Advisers and Geographic Profilers who consider behavioural aspects of crimes.
>
> Professionals require knowledge of investigations as well as a detailed understanding of behaviour.

What is Behavioural Analysis?

There has been an abundance of media attention to **offender profiling**, both in fiction and 'true crime' documentaries on live or cold (historic) cases.

Offender Profiling. Identifying behavioural characteristics of an offender based upon analysis of the crime.

Although pen portraits of offenders had been recognised previously, the work of Brussel (1955) profiling the 'mad bomber', and research undertaken by the Federal Bureau of Investigation (FBI) interviewing and classifying sexual homicide offenders (Ressler, Burgess & Douglas, 1988) – as dramatised in the series Mindhunter (see further reading) brought the practice to notice. In the UK the work of David Canter has highlighted the importance

DOI: 10.4324/9781003431213-15

of **investigative psychology** and scientific rigour in such research – for example considering the use of A→C equations to

Investigative Psychology. Application of psychology to the investigation process.

hypothesise how 'actions' in a crime can lead to consideration of 'characteristics' of typical offenders if sufficient theory, argument or evidence exists to support a link between the two (see Canter, 2017).

Originally there was somewhat of an academic/practitioner 'divide' with academics undertaking more statistical and inductive work – researching many crimes for overall patterns and trends and applying these findings to an individual case; and practitioners being somewhat more clinical and deductive – looking at the individual case and providing advice based upon their experience (see Alison et al., 2004). However, both methods are now pragmatically used in combination, sharing the same overall goal of providing accurate and reliable advice to an investigation (see Petherick & Brooks, 2021).

Offender profiling or *"identifying the personality and behavioural characteristics of the offender based upon an analysis of the crime committed"* (Douglas & Burgess, 1986, p. 9) is now a somewhat dated term, with professionals working in the field preferring the label **Behavioural Investigative Advisers (BIAs)** to criminal profilers. Those working with investigations soon recognised

Behavioural Investigative Adviser (BIA). Professional who applies behavioural science to analyse behaviours in serious crime to assist law enforcement agencies.

that while they could assist in terms of providing an 'offender profile', additional behavioural support could also be provided to police.

Yet it is not only BIAs who undertake behavioural analysis. Detectives consider behavioural features relating to what is sometimes coined as the '5WH': motivation (why), crime location and exit routes (where), modus operandi (how) and time of day (when) to identify the offender (who). **Crime analysts** and researchers look for patterns in offending, and **Geographic Profilers** consider locations of crimes – all providing advice and suggestions

Crime Analysts. Use data to identify patterns and trends in crime.
Geographic Profilers. Analyse offence locations to provide geographic recommendations regarding an offender.

to investigations in relation to who/where to prioritise resources.

How Does Behavioural Analysis Assist the Police?

As noted in Chapter 1, forensic and investigative psychology applies generic psychological theories to a forensic domain. When attempting to identify an offender, an analyst or BIA may utilise knowledge of research into the (un) reliability of some aspects of memory for example. See Box 11.1.

Box 11.1   Applications in real life: Hypothetical use of offender description.

A white female victim aged 18 years was pushed to the floor and sexually assaulted. She described the offender as male, white, 18–20 years, 6 feet tall, medium build, with a gold tooth.

The most reliable feature of this description is likely to be the presence of a gold tooth as we encode, retain and more accurately recall distinguishing features which capture our attention. In addition, as the victim and offender are the same ethnicity – this description is (more) likely to be correct (see Brigham et al., 2007; Johnson, 1983). Moreover, presuming the victim associates with people of a similar age to herself, based on exposure, her age estimation of the male, is also (more) likely to be reliable (see Rhodes & Anastasi, 2012). However, as the victim was pushed to the floor and dependant on the clothes the offender was wearing, her appraisal of height and build may be less accurate (see Loftus, 1996).

As such when releasing descriptive details to the media, constructing a profile or searching dental records or suspect databases, it would be pertinent to consider the offender is *likely* to be white male with a gold or unusual tooth, and *look like* he is in his late teens/early 20s; yet unwise to prioritise people of interest based on their height or build.

Such application of theories/methods are undertaken in a variety of bespoke policing roles.

Behavioural investigative advice

Behavioural Investigative Advisers are generally employed in centralised departments (e.g., FBI USA; National Crime Agency UK), advising on serious, serial and stranger offences such as murder and rape. One reason for these types of offences is they provide the richest level of data/variables. Comparing an armed robbery with a rape, in the former there are few variables, and most offenders act in similar ways. Most wear a balaclava/disguise, break into a bank/somewhere with high value goods, possess a firearm, use threats and escape in a vehicle. Conversely rape offences involve a variety of locations, different sexual activity, weapons (or not), theft (or not), speech (or not) and vehicles (or not). The choices the offender makes can provide clues to the type of person responsible. The more decisions made, the more traits revealed.

Some services provided by BIAs are discussed, but for a full description of other services and discussion of the related forensic clinical psychologist (FCP) work in this field, see Brown et al. (2015) and Sigurdardóttir et al. (2023, 2024).

Offender profile: Part of the BIA role is to provide a profile of an unknown offender to assist the investigation suggesting the type of person most likely to have committed the crime/s using databases of past cases, research and experience. While profiling cannot predict with certainty who committed the offence, the probable type of person more likely to be responsible can be prioritised. Advice has now veered away from the **naïve trait approach**; giving lists of potential traits is theoretically flawed (see Alison et al., 2002) and prac-

Naïve Trait Approach. Predicting personality characteristics from crime scene actions.

tically unusable. Now profiles are pragmatic – utilising information the investigation already has or can easily obtain to identify or prioritise suspects. This can include demographic (e.g., gender, ethnicity, age) and investigative (e.g., previous convictions) information; rather than psychologically interesting, but less identifiable traits (e.g., egocentric, antisocial, sadistic), behaviours (e.g., cruelty to animals) or histories (e.g., severe head injury when young).

DNA screening: If there is DNA (e.g., blood, semen) left at a crime scene which it is believed belongs to the offender, in the UK it may be tested against the National DNA Database of offenders. However, if there is no match to a person, individuals can be 'swabbed' to see if the DNA belongs to them. Who to swab can be prioritised using the offender profile. So, if the profile suggests the offender is likely to be a white male aged 20–30 years living in a certain district – these individuals can be swabbed first to test for a match.

Crime scene assessment (CSA): These assessments can be undertaken by different people – e.g., detectives, when deciding to collect statements, consider whether houses overlook the scene;

Crime Scene Assessment (by BIAs). Evaluation of crime scene actions and choices to consider what is likely to have happened at the scene.

Crime Scene Investigators consider where fingerprints may be located. Also, BIAs conduct a CSA considering the interaction between the offender and victim, the decisions made and potential hypotheses of what is likely to have happened. Box 11.2 details a hypothetical example.

Box 11.2   Applications in real life: Hypothetical CSA of a murder.

A female body is found stabbed several times, with her hands bound behind her back. There is no evidence of sexual activity, but her purse (containing cash and cards) and phone are missing. These are not believed to have been subsequently used. The CCTV has captured a potential suspect following the female victim out of a nightclub, dashcam evidence from passing cars trace the suspect as he/she follows her down a street, and several camera doorbells see them pass through a housing estate. The victim tried ringing a friend who did not pick up. At the end of the housing estate is a park where the victim's body was found.

A BIA conducting a CSA would consider the decisions made by the offender – why was she not attacked outside the club, on the road or in the housing estate? Why was her body left where it would easily be found? Consideration is taken of all potential options the offender had, and decisions made. Did she know her attacker hence why they stole the phone? Was this for monetary or personal value? Why were her hands tied – were bindings sexually motivated, used as torture, or to control her resistance? Consideration of what happened and why – to compare the likelihood of different hypotheses, can assist in generation and prioritisation of potential lines of investigative enquiry.

Case Linkage Analysis: If more than one similar crime has occurred but there is no forensic evidence (such as DNA) to link them, a BIA can consider which

Case Linkage Analysis. Consideration of whether a potential series of offences are linked to one or more offenders.

offences may be linked i.e., is there a serial offender? While the process of offence linkage is somewhat complex (see Woodhams & Bennell, 2014) it involves consideration of the behavioural similarities and differences between the crimes, in conjunction with the frequency of behaviours. For example, offences occurring in close geographic proximity to one another, involving rare behaviours – are more likely to be linked, than offences occurring far apart with more frequent behaviours shown – see Box 11.3.

Box 11.3   Applications in real life: Hypothetical offence linkage.

Two sex offences have occurred in a small town, two weeks apart. In both the offender is wearing a pink balaclava, victims' hands are tied with a ribbon, and they are threatened with a crossbow. Owing to the proximity of the offences and the unusual (distinctive) behaviours displayed – these offences may be linked – i.e., are likely to have been committed by the same offender.

Two sex offences have occurred in January and September of the same year – one in Exeter, Devon, the other in Edinburgh, Scotland. In both, the offender is wearing a plain black baseball cap and tells the victim to 'shut up'. Owing to the fact that these offences are 400+ miles apart and temporally distant, many people wear black baseball caps, and telling victims to 'shut up' is common; they are less likely to be linked.

Crime analysis

Crime analysts look for patterns between offences, and inconsistencies in information (College of Policing, 2025). There are a range of roles – for example the Serious Crime Analysis Section analyses serious crimes of murder, rape and abduction – to identify potential serial offenders in the UK. Conversely analysts working in individual police forces may produce **problem profiles** which give an understanding of established or emerging crime locally, noting 'hotspots' or specific areas of offending to enable deployment of resources. They may focus

Problem Profiles. An understanding of an established or emerging crime or issue.

on key individuals –
providing detailed **sub-
ject profiles** on victims'
or offenders' demo-
graphic information, or
summaries of victimisa-
tion/offending to assist
in protecting victims or
apprehending offend-

Subject Profile. Detailed report
regarding an offender or victim.
Charting Associations. Visual dia-
grams that map out relationships
between individuals, locations,
events, and criminal activities.

ers. They also look in depth at suspects/groups – analysing phone,
social media and financial transactions, and developing **charting
associations**. Analysts use data to make valid inferences and provide recommendations for prevention and deployment, and to
guide future strategies (College of Policing, 2025).

Geographic profiling

Stemming from environmental psychology and the work of practitioners such as Kim Rossmo (Rossmo, 1999) and academics like
David Canter (e.g. Canter, 2007), geographic profiling can be
undertaken as a bespoke role or by considering geographic principles in analysis. Geographic profiling focusses on time and location, incorporating theories such as routine activity (see Chapter 5)
to consider when and where people offend. This can highlight
locations an offender
may live at or have
some kind of **anchor**
with (e.g., previous
association, workplace,
leisure). It can be used
in a variety of offences

Anchor. Location in which the
offender has some association e.g.,
residence, workplace, leisure.

(see for example Kocsis & Irwin, 1997), in a variety of ways, to
prioritise areas. This can lead to investigative suggestions regarding prioritisation of suspects, where to deploy covert cameras or
where an offender may have buried a body for example.

A Note of Caution

It is important to recognise that professionals working in these
roles require not only behavioural, but also investigative knowledge for their advice to be of use – see Box 11.4.

Box 11.4   Case study: Murder of Rachel Nickell.

A psychologist provided advice to the murder investigation of 23-year-old Rachel Nickell in London. His profile stated the offender would be lonely, socially incompetent, and have certain sexual fantasies (Britton, 1997). A suspect was identified, and an undercover operation was devised to see if he would divulge fantasies aligning to those predicted. Colin Stagg was deemed to fit the profile, having a *"sexually deviant-based personality disturbance"* (Bennetto, 2002), and charged for the murder. At court, the evidence was deemed inadmissible and the defendant found not guilty. Mr Justice Ognall described the *'honey trap'* used as showing *"excessive zeal"*. The psychologist faced professional scrutiny, although a disciplinary hearing for professional misconduct by the British Psychological Society collapsed after eight years (Morris, 2002).

While the Senior Investigative Officer in a case holds overall responsibility for investigative decisions, the controversy fuelled the need for 'behavioural' advisers to also have 'investigative' knowledge of policies and procedures relating to the rules of evidence. A television adaptation of the case is depicted in Deceit (see further reading) and the interested reader is guided to Ormerod and Sturman (2013).

This example emphasises that although behavioural analysis can influence investigations, it may prove counter-productive if not applied in conjunction with investigative knowledge – a detailed understanding of interview protocols, court requirements, rules of disclosure and the like, which general psychological training does not provide.

Summary

This chapter outlined how behavioural analysis can assist investigations in a variety of ways. Examples highlight the complex nature of the work, and the need for practitioners to have both behavioural and investigative knowledge for valid application.

Further Reading

Websites – The College of Policing website offers detailed information regarding crime analysis in the UK www.college.police.uk/app/intelligence-management/intelligence-products

The National Crime Agency website depicts the work of the Serious Crime Analysis Section www.nationalcrimeagency.gov.uk/what-we-do/how-we-work/providing-specialist-capabilities-for-law-enforcement/serious-crime-analysis?

Videos – The TV dramatisation Mindhunter depicts the pioneering work of the FBI Behavioural Science Unit www.imdb.com/title/tt5290382/

The real story of Ann Burgess' career is told here www.youtube.com/watch?v=VKy6oB2eqJM

A TV dramatisation of the case of Rachel Nickell is found here www.imdb.com/title/tt12994306/%20

Podcasts – "Crime Analyst" podcast by Laura Richards behaviourally dissects cases www.crime-analyst.com

Dara interviews Terri about her role as a BIA www.youtube.com/watch?v=3gzGfdabxjg

Articles – Recent evaluation of the work of UK BIAs and FCPs are detailed here Sigurdardóttir, T. D., Rainbow, L., Gregory, A., Gregory, P., & Gudjonsson, G. H. (2023). The current role and contribution of "behavioural investigative advisers" (BIAs) to criminal investigation in the United Kingdom. *Journal of Criminal Psychology*, *14*(2), 136–156.

Sigurdardóttir, T. D., West, A., & Gudjonsson, G. H. (2024). The current role and contribution of 'forensic clinical psychologists' (FCPs) to criminal investigation in the United Kingdom. *Journal of Criminal Psychology*, *14*(3), 217–239.

References

Alison, L., Bennell, C., Mokros, A., & Ormerod, D. (2002). The personality paradox in offender profiling: A theoretical review of the processes involved in deriving background characteristics from crime scene actions. *Psychology, Public Policy, and Law*, *8*(1), 115.

Alison, L., West, A., & Goodwill, A. (2004). The academic and the practitioner: Pragmatists' views of offender profiling. *Psychology, Public Policy, and Law*, *10*(1–2), 71.

Bennetto, J. (2002, October 28). *Psychologist in Stagg case faces misconduct charge.* The Independent. www.independent.co.uk/news/uk/crime/psychologist-in-stagg-case-faces-misconduct-charge-141253.html

Brigham, J. C., Bennett, L. B., Meissner, C. A., & Mitchell, T. L. (2007). The influence of race on eyewitness memory. In R.C.L. Lindsay, D.F. Ross, J. D. Read & M. P. Toglia (Eds.), *The handbook of eyewitness psychology: Volume II* (pp. 271–296). Psychology Press. https://doi. org/10.4324/9780203936368

Britton, P. (1997. *The jigsaw man.* Random House.

Brown, J., Shell, Y., & Cole, T. (2015). *Forensic psychology.* Routledge.

Brussel, J. (1955). The mad bomber. Casebook of a crime psychiatrist (New English Library (pp. 7–73). In J. Brown (Ed.), *Forensic psychology – Critical concepts in psychology.* Routledge.

Canter, D. (2007). *Mapping murder: The secrets of geographical profiling.* Random House.

Canter, D. (2017). *Criminal psychology.* Routledge.

College of Policing. Retrieved January 27, 2025 from www.college.pol ice.uk/

Douglas, J. E., & Burgess, A. E. (1986). Criminal profiling: A viable investigative tool against violent crime. *FBI Law Enforcement Bulletin,* 55(12), 9–13.

Johnson, S. L. (1983). Cross-racial identification errors in criminal cases. *Cornell Law Review,* 69, 934.

Kocsis, R. N., & Irwin, H. J. (1997). An analysis of spatial patterns in serial rape, arson, and burglary: The utility of the circle theory of environmental range for psychological profiling. *Psychiatry, Psychology and Law,* 4(2), 195–206.

Loftus, E. F. (1996). *Eyewitness testimony.* Harvard University Press.

Morris, S. (2002, October 31). *Honeytrap case collapses.* The Guardian. www.theguardian.com/uk/2002/oct/31/ukcrime.stevenmorris

Ormerod, D., & Sturman, J. (2013). Working with the courts: Advice for expert witnesses. In L. Alison (Ed.), *Forensic psychologists casebook* (pp. 170–193). Willan.

Petherick, W., & Brooks, N. (2021). Reframing criminal profiling: A guide for integrated practice. *Psychiatry, Psychology and Law,* 28(5), 694–710.

Ressler, R. K., Burgess, A. W., & Douglas, J. E. (1988). *Sexual homicide: Patterns and motives.* Lexington Books/D. C. Heath and Com.

Rhodes, M. G., & Anastasi, J. S. (2012). The own-age bias in face recognition: a meta-analytic and theoretical review. *Psychological Bulletin,* 138(1), 146.

Rossmo, D. K. (1999). *Geographic profiling.* CRC press.

Sigurdardóttir, T. D., Rainbow, L., Gregory, A., Gregory, P., & Gudjonsson, G. H. (2023). The current role and contribution of "behavioural investigative advisers" (BIAs) to criminal investigation in the United Kingdom. *Journal of Criminal Psychology,* 14(2), 136–156.

Sigurdardóttir, T. D., West, A., & Gudjonsson, G. H. (2024). The current role and contribution of 'forensic clinical psychologists' (FCPs) to criminal investigation in the United Kingdom. *Journal of Criminal Psychology*, *14*(3), 217–239.

Woodhams, J., & Bennell, C. (Eds.). (2014). *Crime linkage: Theory, research, and practice*. CRC press.

Chapter 12

Interviewing Suspects

Key Points

Many suspects deny involvement in crimes even when confronted with evidence. Investigative interviewing needs to be effective to secure evidence but also needs to be reliable to prevent wrongful convictions.

Accusatory interviewing approaches such as the Reid Model use interrogation to pressure suspects into confessing. Many argue that such approaches are unethical and contribute to false convictions.

Information-gathering interviewing, as outlined in the PEACE Framework, prioritises truth seeking. While valuing building rapport and transparency it allows for appropriate probing and challenging suspects when inconsistencies are observed.

The Complexity of a Suspect Interview

Interviewing crime suspects presents distinct challenges as they are more likely to deceive and less likely to cooperate compared witnesses (Arnold, 2021). The outcomes of these interviews significantly influence subsequent police actions, including charging decisions and court evidence (Haworth, 2020). Ineffective suspect interviews can result in guilty parties evading justice, wasted resources, and wrongful convictions (Gudjonsson, 2021). The Innocence Project estimates that 25% of exonerated prisoners had falsely confessed to a crime

DOI: 10.4324/9781003431213-16

they had not committed (Innocence Project, n.d.). As exemplified in Box 12.1, many false confessions can be attributed to ineffective and unreliable interviewing methods (Gudjonsson, 2021) – unsurprising given that some reports suggest many officers receive inadequate on-the-job training on suspect interviews (Cleary & Warner, 2016). Law enforcement should adopt effective, evidence-based interviewing strategies. Two interviewing methods commonly used today include **accusatory approaches** and **information-gathering approaches**.

Accusatory approach interviewing. Suspect interrogation that assumes guilt and prioritises eliciting a confession, often through coercive techniques.

Information gathering approach interviewing. Investigative interviewing approach that prioritises information gathering over eliciting confessions, typically using rapport-building and active listening techniques.

Box 12.1   Case study: The Central Park Five (Ryan, 2002; Smith, 2002)

On 19 April 1989, a female jogger was raped in Central Park, Manhattan. Various groups of teenagers entered the park that night, with numerous reports of muggings and assaults. Six black teenagers, 14–16 years, were witnessed in the park, and brought in for questioning. Each suspect was interrogated and subjected to intense questioning without a solicitor. No interrogations were recorded, and the teenagers later explained they were coerced, lied to, and intimidated into providing false confessions. For example, one suspect was falsely informed by the detective that his fingerprints were on the victim's clothes, leading him to admitting being at the crime scene. Resultingly five of the six teenagers admitted they were accomplices while the others conducted the rape. Despite all five recanting their confessions a few weeks later, they were all convicted on multiple charges including assault, robbery, and rape; their sentences ranging between seven and 13 years. Over a decade later the convictions were overturned when an incarcerated serial rapist (Matias Reyes) confessed to being the culprit, substantiated through DNA evidence. As well as drawing attention to ongoing issues with racial profiling and discrimination, this high-profile case is one of many highlighting the problems with unreliable and unethical suspect interviewing techniques.

The Accusatory Approach

Accusatorial interrogation techniques operate on the presumption of guilt, focusing on eliciting confessions rather than determining innocence (Meissner et al., 2014). As such, this approach is considered as an evidence (of guilt) gathering process, rather than an investigative interview. **The Reid model** is one of the most widely-known interrogative frameworks, widely adopted by North American investigators since the 1940s (Inbau et al., 2013; Pozzulo et al., 2013). This high-pressure, coercive interviewing strategy comprises of nine steps (see Box 12.2) which use maximisation and minimisation techniques to make a confession appear the most appealing option for the suspect (Kassin, 2014; Kassin et al., 2010). **Maximisation techniques** serve to increase the suspect's belief in an inevitable conviction through grand accusations, presenting evidence, and limiting defence opportunities (Kassin, 2014). **Minimisation techniques** encourage confessions by reducing the perceived severity

The Reid model. An accusatory interviewing method that aims to elicit a confession through minimisation and maximisation techniques.

Maximisation techniques. Psychological techniques designed to elicit a confession through presenting conviction as an inevitable outcome.

of the crime, showing sympathy or understanding, and creating a false sense of leniency (Kassin, 2014; Kassin et al., 2010).

Minimisation techniques. Psychological techniques designed to elicit a confession by reducing the suspect's perceived severity of the crime.

Criticisms

The Reid technique's confrontational nature and focus on guilt acceptance make it effective in securing confessions, contributing to its popularity. However, the accuracy of these confessions is questionable (King & Snook, 2009), with many arguing its coercive nature can result in false confessions (Gudjonsson & Pearse, 2011). Research indicates guilt-presumptive interrogations are more likely to produce confessions, regardless of their truthfulness (Areh, 2016). This is partly due to **confirmation bias**, where investigators favour

Confirmation bias. Tendency to search for, interpret or favour evidence in support of one's existing beliefs.

information supporting their belief in the suspect's guilt while disregarding contradictory evidence (see further discussion of biases in Chapter 13). Consequently, there is significant concern over the reliability of confessions obtained through accusatorial methods like the Reid model (Kassin, 2014; Salvati & Houck, 2019). Additionally, other coercive tactics, such as feigning friendship, appealing to religious beliefs, and presenting false evidence, have been found to manipulate individuals into providing false confessions (Gudjonsson, 2001; Kassin, 2014). Overall, confession-seeking interviews can harm suspects, damage the reputation of investigating agencies, and erode public trust in the criminal justice system (Cleary & Bull, 2019; Etienne & McAdams, 2021; Sivasubramaniam & Heuer, 2012), as well as potentially leading to the actual offenders not being apprehended and left loose in the community to commit further crimes.

Box 12.2   The Reid Model (Inbau et al., 2013)

1. **Direct positive confrontation**: Interviewer immediately accuses the suspect of committing the offence in a confident and assertive manner. Suspect is advised it would be in their best interest to admit guilt early on.

2. **Theme development**: Interviewer demonstrates an understanding of the suspect and uses this to develop a theme around why they committed their offence. E.g., showing an understanding of their motivation, normalising or minimising the seriousness, or justifying their behaviour.

3. **Handling denials:** Interviewers interrupt suspects every time they attempt to deny accusations.

4. **Overcoming objections**: The suspect is likely to make objections supporting their innocence (e.g., "*I could never have done that, I am not a violent person*"). Interviewers are advised to use this to further develop motive (e.g., "*so it must have been a spur of the moment thing*").

5. **Procurement and retention of the suspect's attention:** Many suspects will focus on the punishment faced hence act defensively. Interviewers should intensify the discussion, physically getting into closer proximity, and use gestures to show an understanding of the suspect's reasons for offending.

6. **Handle the suspect's passive mood:** The interviewer is required to intensify discussions into motivation, whilst still demonstrating sympathy.

7. **Presenting an alternative question**: The interviewer presents the suspect with two scenarios of how the offence unfolded. Though both accuse the suspect, one is considerably worse in relation to immorality and repercussions. As a result, the suspect is encouraged to confess to the least problematic scenario, although they could deny both scenarios.

8. **Orally relate details of the offence**: Once the suspect accepts one of the scenarios, the investigator must follow it with a statement of reinforcement. Further questions

should be asked to get a more complete confession and information about their method of offending and motive.

9. **Convert the oral confession into a written confession:** Information from step 8 is used to create a written confession the suspect is required to sign.

The Information Gathering Approach

The negative outcomes associated with accusatory interrogations have given preference to the use of information-gathering approaches which prioritise obtaining a truthful account from the suspect rather than merely seeking a confession (Eastwood & Watkins, 2021). This approach involves *interviewing rather than interrogating*, aiming to elicit information about the crime from the suspect's perspective without presuming guilt (Bull, 2023). Consequently, information-gathering interviews are less confrontational and do not impose coercive tactics. Evidence from empirical research shows greater support towards the use of such approaches. A meta-analysis suggests information-gathering approaches reduce the risk of false confessions without reducing the frequency of truthful confessions (Meissner et al., 2012, 2014), presenting this approach as a more reliable and ethical method for suspect interviews.

A prominent information gathering approach model is the PEACE framework, which can be used for interviewing suspects, witnesses and victims. The approach was developed in England during the early 1990s in response to concerns about coercive interviews and false confessions (Milne et al., 2007). It was informed by initial evaluations of pre-recorded suspect interviews. Professor John Baldwin highlighted problematic interviewing strategies such as poor preparation, repetitive questioning (to encourage a different response), and psychological pressure (as used in accusatory interviews).

The PEACE framework is a systematic five-step approach

PEACE framework. Information-gathering interview technique that is non-accusatory and focusses on rapport building and transparency.

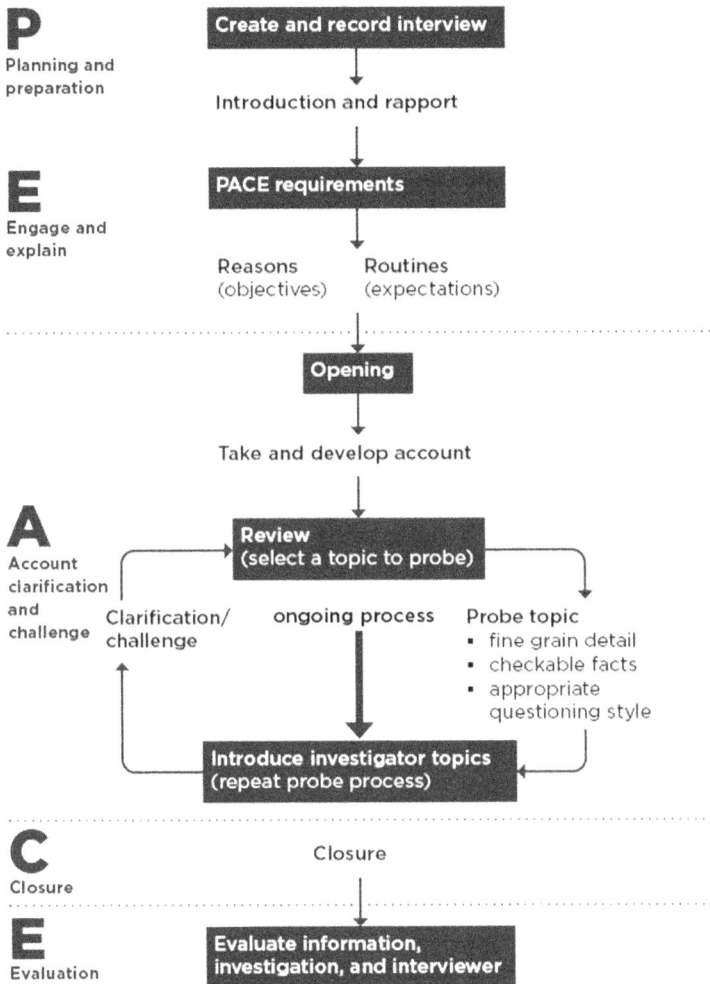

Figure 12.1 PEACE framework.

(Figure 12.1) which aims to ensure ethical, transparent, and reliable investigative interviews (Clarke et al., 2011). The first component requires investigators to carefully *Plan and Prepare* the interview in advance, reviewing the evidence and setting out their objectives. Following this, the *Engage and Explain* component centres around establishing rapport with the interviewee and explaining the purpose and expectations of the interview. A central tenet of the main information gathering process (*Account, Clarification, and Challenge*) is to treat the interview as conversation management, focusing on gathering reliable information ethically rather than using coercive techniques such as deception, intimidation and pressure (Adam & van Golde, 2019). However, investigators are required to review the information provided, probe for further information and challenge them on any inconsistencies. During the *Closure* stage, investigators will summarise the interview and confirm key points with the interviewee; and after the interview has concluded, *Evaluation* – review the interview and consider subsequent actions needed (e.g., if further questioning is required).

Evaluation

Since its inception, PEACE has been adopted by law enforcement worldwide, including agencies in Australia, Canada, and New Zealand (Adam & van Golde, 2019; Dixon, 2010; Schollum, 2005). The model has proven effective in reducing false confessions and improving the quality of interviews (Clark & Milne, 2001; Cunningham, 2010; Milne & Bull, 2003; Moston, 2009; Scott et al., 2015). The framework necessitates training, ensuring users are well-versed in effective interviewing methods and to maintain consistency (De Vito, 2008; Silverman et al., 2008). However, the effectiveness of PEACE training in improving interview quality remains debated. Griffiths and Milne (2006) found training enhanced officers' interviewing skills, but some communication skills diminished after a year. Walsh and Milne (2008) evaluated PEACE training and found 31% of fraud investigators were rated as skilled or highly skilled, compared to only 6% of untrained investigators, however the training did not significantly improve *preparation and planning* skills or the *engage and explain* stage. Clarke et al. (2011) found no significant differences between trained and untrained interviewers in interviewing efficacy, however, workplace supervision improved performance at the *engage and explain* stage. These findings highlight the importance of high-quality, continuous training for the PEACE framework (Walsh & Milne, 2008) and a greater understanding of specific features within it.

Summary

This chapter reviewed two distinct approaches to suspect interviews. The accusatory approach could appear as a more favorable approach due to its focus on confessions, however, it involves unethical practices and creates a higher risk of false confessions. Information-gathering approaches like the PEACE framework are increasingly adopted, replacing coercive methods though some academics argue such interviews still contain a variety of psychological persuasion tactics underlying its success. While academics generally favour the ethical, transparent, and reliable PEACE framework, many practitioners (namely from North America) still support accusatory methods in contexts where deception is anticipated, and public safety necessitates a utilitarian perspective (Miller et al., 2018).

Further Reading

Video – Emily and Laurence Alison on Rapport:
www.youtube.com/watch?v=RGfEWeSO82g
Web page – College of Policing (England & Wales) page detailing professional practise around Investigative Interviewing (including PEACE framework):   www.college.police.uk/app/investigation/investigative-interviewing/investigative-interviewing
Podcast – "The Reid Technique and the Wrongful Conviction of Darrel Parker" by *Crimes of the Centuries.*

References

Adam, L., & van Golde, C. (2020). Police practice and false confessions: A search for the implementation of investigative interviewing in Australia. *Alternative Law Journal, 45*(1), 52–59. https://doi.org/10.1177/1037969X19874415

Areh, I. (2016). Police interrogations through the prism of science. *Psiholoska Obzorja, 25*(1), 18–28. doi:10.20419/2016.25.440

Arnold, L. (2021). Strategies used by suspects during a police interview [PhD thesis, University of Portsmouth]. Portsmouth, UK.

https://pure.port.ac.uk/ws/portalfiles/portal/28231006/Lucy_A rnold_Thesis_Final_May_2021.pdf

Bull, R. (2023). Improving the interviewing of suspects using the PEACE model: A comprehensive overview. *Canadian Journal of Criminology and Criminal Justice*, 65(1), 80–91. https://doi.org/10.3138/cjccj.2023-0003

Clarke, C., & Milne, R. (2001). National evaluation of the PEACE investigative interviewing course: Project Report 149 (Police Research Award Scheme), i–ii.

Clarke, C., Milne, R., & Bull, R. (2011). Interviewing suspects of crime: The impact of PEACE training, supervision and the presence of a legal advisor. *Journal of Investigative Psychology and Offender Profiling*, 8(2), 149–162. https://doi.org/10.1002/jip.144

Cleary, H. M., & Bull, R. (2019). Jail inmates' perspectives on police interrogation. *Psychology, Crime & Law*, 25(2), 157–170. https://doi.org/10.1080/1068316X.2018.1503667

Cleary, H., & Warner, T. C. (2016). Police training in interviewing and interrogation methods: A comparison of techniques used with adult and juvenile suspects. *Law and Human Behavior*, 40(3), 270.

Cunningham, S. (2010). *Evaluation of the Implementation of Investigative Interviewing Training and Assessment (Level 1) Final Report*. New Zealand Police.

De Vito, J. A. (2008). *Messages: Building interpersonal communication skills*. Allyn & Bacon.

Dixon, D. (2010, October 22). Interrogating Myths: A comparative study of practices, research, and regulation. Research Paper No 2010–40, UNSW Law. https://papers.ssrn.com/sol3/papers.cfm?abstract_id¼1689358.

Eastwood, J., & Watkins, K. (2021). Psychological persuasion in suspect interviews: Reid, PEACE, and pathways forward. *Investigative Interviewing: Research & Practice*, 11(1),54.

Etienne, M., & McAdams, R. (2021). Police deception in interrogation as a problem of procedural legitimacy. *Texas Tech Law Review*, 54, 21.

Griffiths, A., & Milne, R. (2006). Will it all end in tiers? Police interviews with suspects in Britain. In T. Williamson (Ed.), *Investigative interviewing: Rights, research, regulation* (pp. 167–189). Willan.

Gudjonsson, G. (2001). False confession. *Psychologist*, 14(11), 588–559.

Gudjonsson, G. H. (2021). The science-based pathways to understanding false confessions and wrongful convictions. *Frontiers in Psychology*, 12, https://doi.org/10.3389/fpsyg.2021.633936

Gudjonsson, G. H., & Pearse, J. (2011). Suspect interviews and false confessions. *Current Directions in Psychological Science*, 20(1), 33–37. https://doi.org/10.1177/0963721410396824

Haworth, K. (2020). Police interviews in the judicial process: Police interviews as evidence. In M. Coulthard, A. May & R. Sousa-Silva (Eds.), *The Routledge handbook of forensic linguistics* (pp. 144–158). Routledge. https://doi.org/10.4324/9780429030581

Inbau, F. E., Reid, J. E., Buckley, J. P., & Jayne, B. C. (2013). *Essentials of the Reid technique: Criminal interrogation and confessions.* Jones & Bartlett Publishers.

Innocence Project. (n.d.). False Confessions or Admissions. Retrieved March 24, 2018, from www.innocenceproject.org/causes/false-conf essions- admissions/

Kassin, S. M. (2014). False confessions: Causes, consequences, and implications for reform. *Policy Insights from the Behavioral and Brain Sciences, 1*(1), 112–121. doi:10.1177/ 2372732214548678

Kassin, S. M., Appleby, S. C., & Perillo, J. T. (2010). Interviewing suspects: Practice, science, and future directions. *Legal and Criminological Psychology, 15*(1), 39–55. https://doi.org/10.1348/135532509 X449361

King, L., & Snook, B. (2009). Peering inside a Canadian interrogation room: An examination of the Reid model of interrogation, influence tactics, and coercive strategies. *Criminal Justice and Behavior, 36*(7), 674–694. https://doi.org/10.1177/0093854809335142

Meissner, C. A., Redlich, A. D., Bhatt, S., & Brandon, S. (2012). Interview and interrogation methods and their effects on true and false confessions. *Campbell Systematic Reviews, 8*(1), 1–53. https://doi. org/10.4073/csr.2012.13

Meissner, C. A., Redlich, A. D., Michael, S. W., Evans, J. R., Camilletti, C. R., Bhatt, S., & Brandon, S. (2014). Accusatorial and information-gathering interrogation methods and their effects on true and false confessions: A meta-analytic review. *Journal of Experimental Criminology, 10*(4), 459–486. https://doi.org/10.1007/s11292-014-9207-6

Milne, R., & Bull, R. (2003). Interviewing by the police. In D. Carson & R. Bull (Eds.), *Handbook of psychology in legal contexts* (p. 111). Wiley.

Milne, R., Shaw, G., & Bull, R. (2007). Investigative interviewing: The role of research. In D. Carson, R. Milne, F. Pakes, K. Shaley & A. Shawyer (Eds.), *Applying psychology to criminal justice* (p. 67). Wiley.

Miller, J. C., Redlich, A. D., & Kelly, C. E. (2018). Accusatorial and information-gathering interview and interrogation methods: A multi-country comparison. *Psychology, Crime & Law, 24*(9), 935–956. https://doi.org/10.1080/1068316X.2018.1467909

Moston, S. (2009). Investigative interviewing in Australia. In T. Williamson, B. Milne & S. Savage (Eds.), *International developments in investigative interviewing* (pp. 3–23). Willan Publishing.

Pozzulo, J., Forth, A. E., & Bennell, C. (2013). *Forensic psychology.* Pearson Prentice Hall.

Ryan, N. E. (2002, December 5). *"Affirmation in response to motion to vacate judgment of conviction"* (PDF). Supreme Court of the State of New York, County of New York.

Salvati, J. M., & Houck, S. C. (2019). Examining the causes and consequences of confession-eliciting tactics during interrogation. *Journal of Applied Security Research, 14*(3), 241–256.

Schollum, M. (2005). *Investigative interviewing: The literature* (p. 103). NZ Office of the Commissioner of Police.

Scott, A. J., Tudor-Owen, J., Pedretti, P., & Bull, R. (2015). How intuitive is PEACE? Newly recruited police officers' plans, interviews and self-evaluations. *Psychiatry, Psychology and Law, 22*(3), 355.

Silverman, J., Kurtz, S. M., & Draper, J. (2008) *Skills for communicating with patients* (2 ed.). Radcliffe Publishing Ltd.

Sivasubramaniam, D., & Heuer, L. (2012). Procedural justice evaluations in interrogations. In B. L. Cutler (Ed.), *Conviction of the innocent: Lessons from psychological research* (pp. 79–102). American Psychological Association. https://doi.org/10.1037/13085-004

Smith, C. (2002, October 21). Central Park Revisited. *New York.* Retrieved February 13, 2013.

Walsh, D. W., & Milne, R. (2008). Keeping the PEACE? A study of investigative interviewing practices in the public sector. *Legal and Criminological Psychology, 13*(1), 39–57. DOI: 10.1348/135532506X157179

Chapter 13

Decision Making

Key Points

Decisions are made by various individuals throughout the Criminal Justice System.

There are many theories as to why and how we make decisions including making a rational choice by weighing the pros and cons.

Heuristics and biases can affect the decisions we make.

Making decisions in time constrained, high stake, complex, 'natural' environments can be more difficult.

Considering alternatives, using experts or reviewers and taking more time can enhance decision making.

The Importance of Decision Making in Everyday Life

We all make a multitude of decisions from the moment we wake up – do we have time to snooze the alarm? Do we make lunch or buy it? Do we do our assignment (or write this book!) or go out? Familiar decisions are often automated – like washing our hands before preparing food; and some are time critical – we will immediately stop our vehicle at a red light. There are many types of decisions, occurring in different contexts, with various levels of consequence (snoozing an alarm may be less severe than running a red light). We make decisions which only effect ourselves (not brushing our teeth – unless you are speaking at close range

DOI: 10.4324/9781003431213-17

to others!) or depending on our position – decisions which have far reaching effects on others (those in charge of the nuclear 'red button').

Decision Making in the Criminal Justice System

Throughout the criminal justice system, participants make decisions at different stages – see Table 13.1.

Some decisions require individual choices based on many factors – a victim deciding whether to report an offence may consider features such as who the offender was (e.g., were they known to one another?) and their previous experience/conceptions of police (e.g., can/will they do anything?) Other decisions may be organisational based on guidance – for instance in the UK, police utilise the National Decision Model (College of Policing, 2024), Crown Prosecution Service (CPS) follow the code of conduct (Crown Prosecution Service, 2015), and judges utilise sentencing guidelines (Sentencing Council, 2020). However, early on researchers identified criminal justice as a potentially high-risk area for faulty decision making (Tversky & Kahneman, 1974).

How Do We Make Decisions: Theory

There are many theories surrounding decision making and related concepts of **judgement, reasoning** and **problem solving**. These pertain to comparisons between decisions taken by experts versus those taken by novices; quick and slower paced decision making, and decisions made in high-stake situations. Some relevant theories surrounding criminal justice are considered here.

Judgement. The final decision based on reasoning and evaluation.
Reasoning. The process of analysing information and drawing conclusions.
Problem Solving. The process of applying reasoning and finding solutions to a problem.

Table 13.1 Summary of Decisions Made Throughout the Criminal Justice Process.

Offender	Victim	Police	Crown Prosecution Service	Jury	Judge
Do I commit a crime? Do I hand myself in to police?	Do I tell someone? Who do I tell?	What actions are required? What resources are available?	What crime has been committed? Do we have enough evidence?	Do I understand the evidence? Who is telling the truth?	Is the trial being fair to all parties? What disposal is appropriate?
Do I confess?	How can I recover?	Where can we find evidence?	Is it in the public interest to pursue?	Is the suspect guilty?	How long should the sentence be?

Rational choice

One prominent theory regarding how we choose between different options is the **Rational Choice Theory** (Cornish & Clarke, 1986). This suggests that we weigh up the costs and ben-

Rational Choice Theory. Weighing up the costs versus the benefits – deciding upon the best available outcome, with the least potential cost.

efits of each choice, and decide upon the best available outcome, with the least potential cost. For example, a burglar may consider the type of property to target based on risks and reward – outlined in Table 13.2 (also see Nee & Meenaghan, 2006).

While making intuitive sense, in many situations humans act irrationally particularly when emotions are involved. For example, a drug addict may not consider the 'costs' of theft (e.g., criminal record) as their need for money to purchase a fix outweighs rationality.

Heuristics and biases

Instead, we may search for alternative decisions until we find one 'good enough' (satisficing) – our rationality is 'bounded'

Table 13.2 Considerations in Targeting Property.

PROPERTY TYPE			
House		Jewellery shop	
Benefit	Cost	Benefit	Cost
Secluded location	May be occupied	Likely to be empty at night	Alarms, CCTV
Easy entry	Lower yield (phones, cash)	Likely high yield (jewellery)	Difficult entry
Easy to sell, unidentifiable goods			Need bespoke market to sell, identifiable goods

meaning we can settle for less-than-optimal decisions (Simon, 1956). Tversky and Kahneman (1974) detailed predictable **heuristics** we may use, consciously or unconsciously, particularly in circumstances of uncertainty or complexity (see Morvan & Jenkins, 2017). These mental shortcuts/ strategies can be useful to inform decisions, but can lead to unreliable **inferences** as noted in Table 13.3.

Heuristics. Mental shortcuts/ strategies to inform decisions.

Inferences. Conclusions/assumptions made from the available evidence.

When heuristics lead to changes in behaviour they form **biases** – a predisposition to one preference over another, which may be wrong. These too can lead to errors; see Table 13.4.

Biases. Predisposition to one preference over another, which may be wrong.

Some, such as confirmation bias are particularly prominent during emotion provoking events where quick results are required (Ask & Alison, 2010) – as in serious crime investigations.

Table 13.3 How Heuristics Can Lead to Potential Errors.

Heuristic	Description	Examples of potential errors
Anchoring	Being influenced by first impressions	Believing a suspect is guilty based upon a negative first impression
Availability	Attending to information easy to retrieve	After dealing with a false allegation of rape, an investigator thinks a subsequent victim is lying
Representativeness	Over-attending to salient information	Believing a witness in court merely because they are smartly dressed

Table 13.4 How Biases Can Lead to Potential Errors.

Bias	Description	Examples of potential errors
Confirmation	Searching for evidence to confirm preconceptions	An investigation focusses all attention on one suspect they believe responsible to the detriment of other persons of interest ('Tunnel vision' – see Findley & Scott, 2006)
Authority	Favouring authority figures' input over others	Believing a witness account merely because they are a 'Dr'
Conformity	Making a decision based on the majority (groupthink)	A juror being swayed by the other jurors' decisions ('Jury Think' – see Lybrand, Dobson & Solomon, n.d.)
Over-confidence	Favouring those who act with confidence	Believing a witness who articulates they are 'sure'
Feature positive effect	Focussing only on the benefits of the decision	Encouraging a victim to report an offence to the police without consideration of the broader impact on them

Naturalistic decision making (NDM)

Researchers have specifically considered how people make decisions in 'real world' environments. Naturalistic decision making includes decisions made under pressure, in emotive situations, with abundant information (i.e., high cognitive load), where it is unlikely the decision maker has full knowledge of the facts (i.e., uncertainty), and in situations which can change rapidly and which are often unpredictable (see Phillips-Wren & Adya, 2020). Here rather than generating and comparing options, professionals use prior experience to recognise situations quickly, generate solutions, and make

Naturalistic Decision Making (NDM). How people make decisions in complex 'real world' environments.

decisions (Klein, 2008). Difficulties in making decisions in **critical incidents** when there is limited prior experience have also been explored (Shortland et al., 2020).

Critical Incidents. Sudden, potentially dangerous incident, the consequences of which could result in serious harm or significantly impact on public confidence.

How Do We Make Decisions: Practice

Many decisions may not be clear cut in criminal justice environments with time constraints, heuristics, biases and different opinions often involved, exemplified in Boxes 13.1 and 13.2.

Box 13.1 Case study: Murders of Sian O'Callaghan and Becky Godden.

Sian O'Callaghan was reported missing on her way home from a night out in Swindon on 20 March 2011. She was seen on CCTV getting into a taxi belonging to Cristopher Halliwell. An operation was undertaken to follow Halliwell to see if he would lead the investigation to her. He was witnessed purchasing a significant amount of paracetamol to potentially commit suicide, so was arrested. Utilising police kidnap guidance Halliwell was questioned on site, without legal representation.

However, Halliwell confessed to killing Sian and asked the senior investigator if he wanted 'another one'. Detective Superintendent Steve Fulcher agreed, and Halliwell led them to a field where they discovered another body – of missing teenager, Becky Godden.

Despite finding her body at the location supplied, Halliwell's confession was deemed legally inadmissible. At the time there was no imminent risk to (Becky's) life, and correct procedure would have been to caution Halliwell, return him to the police station and question him with legal representation (Police and Criminal Evidence Act,

1984). However, doing so would have run significant risk – Halliwell would (or would be advised to) say 'no comment' and Becky's body would never be found.

Detective Superintendent Fulcher had an ethical, moral and professional dilemma – potentially solve another murder, providing closure to a victim's family; or follow correct procedure and risk never finding her. He chose the former and while highly praised by Becky's family, eventually lost his job over his handling of the case. He said "*I remain convinced that the action that I took in allowing Halliwell to take me to the bodies of both Sian and Becky, was the right and moral thing to do. In so doing, I felt that I correctly prioritised the human rights of the victims and their families, balanced against the rights of the perpetrator*" (Fulcher, 2016). He subsequently wrote a book (Fulcher, 2017), and TV series, A Confession, was a dramatisation of the case.

Halliwell was eventually found guilty of the murder of Becky after new evidence was uncovered.

Box 13.2   Applications in real life: Assessing an offender's fitness to plea.

Forensic psychologist Kerry Daynes (2022) describes case examples of difficult decisions she made when assessing forensic clients. Here she portrays 'Micheal'.

Micheal was accused of the murder of one male and attempted murder of another but had pled guilty to the lesser crimes of manslaughter and attempted manslaughter. The CPS had to decide whether to accept these pleas meaning he could be sentenced without a lengthy (expensive) trial. For acceptance it must be shown that the defendant displayed an 'abnormality of mind' which 'substantially impaired' his responsibility at the time. Although their specific diagnosis differed, four psychiatrists agreed he had been acting on delusional beliefs and auditory hallucinations, concluding he was not culpable for his actions (and therefore should be detained in a psychiatric hospital). However, a fifth psychiatrist disagreed, therefore Kerry was brought in. She states "*it is not unusual for opinions regarding a defendant's mental state to be fiercely contested*" (p. 23), her "*task was to evaluate Micheal's mental state at the ... time of his offences. But months had passed ... there are no medical tests that can confirm the presence or absence of a 'mental illness' ... I had come prepared with an interview schedule and a host of mental health-related questionnaires and personality rating scales ... Given that these phenomena are fleeting, intangible and open to interpretation ... Determining who is and who is not 'normal' is a contentious business ... One of the obvious problems with this type of assessment is that I am largely ... reliant on what a person chooses to share with me. A defendant in a murder case has every incentive not to tell me the full story ... I wanted to question Micheal further ... but I didn't have the rapport ... or the time. My brief was very clear ... circumstances at the time of the offences.*" (pp. 24 – 36).

After six hours (two visits) with Micheal she had two weeks to analyse the data and write a 47-page report. She concluded he had a case for diminished responsibility.

As can be seen in these examples such decisions can significantly affect both the decision maker (personal responsibility, reputation), and others (sentencing). It has been noted that miscarriages of justice can often be traced to poor decision making at some stage (Ask & Fahsing, 2018), and police officers' reasoning and decision making need to be improved (Irving & Dunningham, 1993).

How Can We Improve Decision Making?

There are ways in which decision making can be improved, if implemented. For example:

- using peer review/policy files/logs of decisions – learning from feedback and reflecting upon mistakes
- utilising experts or those with more experience who quickly know which information to focus upon and relevant options (see Knabe-Nicol et al., 2011)
- considering alternative decisions

- not mistaking opinions for facts
- being aware of heuristics and biases
- taking time to decide – slower decisions may be more rational (Kahneman, 2012), however also knowing when to act and when to wait (for a discussion on **decision inertia** see Power & Alison, 2018)
- mixing teams with complimentary skills – e.g., place someone who is willing to make difficult decisions with someone who is thorough and reflective (see Ask & Fahsing, 2018).

> **Decision Inertia.** Tendency to not make or delay decisions or merely repeat previous decisions in new circumstances.

Summary

This chapter considered complexities of decision making in criminal justice. The impact of decisions may have severe consequences for individuals involved. Deciding whether or not to progress a case is vital for a victim. Also, whether a suspect is found guilty or innocent, sentenced in the community or sent to prison – could be life changing. The next two chapters expand upon decisions of forensic psychologists – in relation to assessment and treatment of offenders.

Further Reading

Websites – The UK College of Policing website offers detailed information regarding decision making www.college.police.uk/app/national-decision-model/national-decision-model

The UK CPS code of conduct www.cps.gov.uk/publication/cps-code-conduct and Sentencing guidelines for judges can be found here www.sentencingcouncil.org.uk/sentencing-and-the-council/sentencing-code/

Videos – The investigation into the murders of Sian O'Callaghan and Becky Godden is dramatised in the series 'A Confession' www.imdb.com/title/tt9131050/ with an update on the case and footage of the offender www.youtube.com/watch?v=GetIYi9wd9w

Laurence Alison discusses decision inertia here www.youtube.com/watch?v=nK6R0JoD_dA

Daniel Kahneman discusses his theory of 'thinking fast versus thinking slow' www.youtube.com/watch?v=PirFrDVRBo4

References

Ask, K., & Alison, L. J. (2010). Investigators' decision making. In P. A. Granhag (Ed.), *Forensic psychology in context: Nordic and international perspectives* (pp. 35–55). Willan.

Ask, K., & Fahsing, I. (2018). Investigative decision making. In A. Griffiths, A. & Milne, R. (Eds.) *The psychology of criminal investigation: From theory to practice* (pp. 52–73). Routledge.

College of Policing. (2024). *National Decision Model*. Retrieved 27/01/2025.

Cornish, D., & Clarke, R. V. (1986). *The reasoning criminal: Rational choice perspectives on offending*. Springer- Verlag.

Crown Prosecution Service. (2015). *Code of Conduct*. Retrieved 28/01/2025.

Daynes, K. (2022). *What lies buried: A forensic psychologist's true stories of madness, the bad and the misunderstood*. Endeavour.

Findley, K. A., & Scott, M. S. (2006). Multiple dimensions of tunnel vision in criminal cases. *The Wisconsin Law Rev.*, 291.

Fulcher, S. (2016). Becky Godden detective: Why I broke the rules over Christopher Halliwell. *The Guardian*. 20/09/2016.

Fulcher, S. (2017). *Catching a serial killer: My hunt for murderer Christopher Halliwell, subject of the ITV series A Confession*. Random House.

Irving, B., & Dunningham, C. (1993). *Human factors in the quality control of CID investigations: A brief review of relevant police training*. HM Stationery Office.

Kahneman, D. (2012). *Thinking, fast and slow*. Penguin Books.

Klein, G. (2008). Naturalistic decision making. *Human Factors, 50*(3), 456–460.

Knabe-Nicol, S., Alison, L., & Rainbow, L. (2011). The cognitive expertise of behavioural investigative advisers in the UK and Germany. In L. Alison & L. Rainbow (Eds.), *Professionalizing offender profiling* (pp. 72–125). Routledge.

Lybrand, S., Dobson, J., & Solomon, S. (n.d.). *JuryThink: the social psychology of group deliberation*. DOAR.

Morvan, C., & Jenkins, W. J. (2017). *An analysis of Amos Tversky and Daniel Kahneman's judgment under uncertainty: Heuristics and biases*. Macat Library.

Nee, C., & Meenaghan, A. (2006). Expert decision making in burglars. *British Journal of Criminology, 46*(5), 935–949.

Phillips-Wren, G., & Adya, M. (2020). Decision making under stress: The role of information overload, time pressure, complexity, and uncertainty. *Journal of Decision Systems*, *29*(sup1), 213–225.

Police and Criminal Evidence Act 1984, c. 60. www.legislation.gov.uk/ukpga/1984/60

Power, N., & Alison, L. (2018). Decision inertia in critical incidents. *European Psychologist*.

Sentencing Council. (2020). *Sentencing code*. Retrieved 28/01/2025.

Shortland, N., Alison, L., Thompson, L., Barrett-Pink, C., & Swan, L. (2020). Choice and consequence: A naturalistic analysis of least-worst decision-making in critical incidents. *Memory & Cognition*, *48*, 1334–1345.

Simon, H. A. (1956). Rational choice and the structure of the environment. *Psychological Review*, *63*(2), 129.

Tversky, A., & Kahneman, D. (1974). Judgment under uncertainty: Heuristics and Biases: Biases in judgments reveal some heuristics of thinking under uncertainty. *Science*, *185*(4157), 1124–1131.

Chapter 14

Assessment of Offenders

Key Points

Psychological assessment is used in many domains including forensic psychology.

Many forensic assessments consider the assessment of risk.

Measurements traditionally considered the risk of reoffending.

Measures can be put in place to mitigate and manage risks.

Psychological Assessment

As highlighted by Taylor (2024, p. 127) *"assessment is not a new phenomenon"*. Evaluations of ability, intelligence, personality and thought patterns have been applied in many domains such as measuring suitability for employment.

In the forensic domain there are many reasons for assessments. For example:

- in family court – to assess parents for their suitability to provide appropriate supervision and care of their children
- pre-trial – to determine a suspect's understanding (e.g., did they have the capacity to know they were committing a crime), cognitive functioning (e.g., intelligence, moral development) or mental state (e.g., personality disorders or mental health); or
- post-conviction – to advise an offender's readiness for treatment

DOI: 10.4324/9781003431213-18

Assessment is part of a process which can influence outcomes (e.g., whether parents are granted custody), sentencing (e.g., whether an offender is detained in a secure hospital or prison) and potential treatment. Assessments:

Provide information ... to inform someone – such as a judge, a barrister, a criminal justice team, a forensic mental health team, or an agency – in order to help that person or organisation to make a decision about the individual.

(McGuire & Duff, 2018, p. 403/4).

As such, providing assessments bears a:

Heavy responsibility ... findings can have a significant impact on others' lives.

(Brown, Shell & Cole, 2015, p. 270).

Assessment of offenders involves gathering and evaluating information – collaborating with the individual and seeking **corroborating evidence**. This may involve checking case files, conducting interviews, undertaking a test of abilities

Corroborating Evidence. Supports other evidence (e.g., what is said in interview corroborates what is on file).

(e.g., IQ), assessing mental health (e.g., depression), completing checklists or scales measuring personality types or disorders (e.g., psychopathy), identifying problems (e.g., substance dependence), running physical tests (e.g., plethysmography for measurement of sexual interest) or undertaking neurological assessments (e.g., fMRI for brain imaging). **Psychometric tests** are standardised measures of various constructs or disorders, but their use is highly regulated, and most can only be administered by qualified professionals.

Psychometric Tests. Standardised measures of various constructs or disorders such as ability or personality.

Consideration needs to be given to ethics, usefulness, appropriateness, reliability and the validity of their application, and transparency – which requires that findings are presented back to the individual being assessed. Assessment therefore allows holistic understanding of the person – their background, thoughts, feelings, motivations, attitudes, offending and behaviours –drawing this altogether in **formulation** of the hypotheses about why they have acted. Brown et al. (2015) note that assessments should be individually tailored – however, with limited time, information, and often reluctant clients, the environment is not ideal.

> **Formulation**. Drawing together information to form hypotheses regarding the causes and maintenance of behaviour, to guide treatment.

What is Risk?

Many forensic assessments evaluate the debated concept of 'risk' (Crighton, 2023). Some ponder whether society has become too risk averse – will children soon be climbing trees wearing protective clothing and safety ropes? Or are measures such as wearing helmets when riding bikes necessary? Subjectivity is apparent – bungee jumping may be 'fun' for some, 'foolish' to others. Yet how should acceptable levels of risk be measured, and by whom? Individual decisions based on experience, or statistical measures based on rates of injury? If putting oneself at risk, decisions can be based on individual tolerance; but what if potential risks impact on others' safety? What are acceptable measures of risk to society, and how **reliable** or **valid** are these[1]?

> **Reliable**. Repeated testing will produce similar results.
> **Valid**. A test measures what it claims to.

Risk is considered by different individuals at different stages, for example:

- pre-offence – an offender may weigh the risk versus potential reward of committing a crime

- pre-sentence – a judge may consider risks involved (to the offender and the public) in deciding the type and length of community/custodial sentence
- post-conviction – a psychologist may consider an offender's level of risk before proposing interventions (some only available to high-risk offenders)
- pre-release – a **parole** board will deliberate whether the risk of releasing an offender back into the community is too great (parole denied) or manageable (parole granted but offender is 'managed' with conditions to mitigate potential risk)

> **Parole**. Early release of a prisoner while their sentence is ongoing.

Risk Assessment

Risk assessments evaluate the level of risk, considering the likelihood of something happening (or not). Often a risk assessment is conducted to assess the risk of something bad happening in a certain situation, with mechanisms put in place to reduce that risk. If we are taking a group of students to court for example, we may assess the risk of potential harm and undertake actions to reduce it – see Table 14.1.

> **Risk Assessment**. Evaluates the level of risk, considering the likelihood of something happening (or not).

Risk assessments are increasingly conducted in policing to evaluate the hazards, harm or threat that individuals or situations may pose in order to consider an appropriate response. In forensic practice, risk assessments consider the risk that individuals pose to themselves (e.g., if they are suicidal) or others (e.g., if they previously displayed violence towards others) under certain conditions (e.g., in specific situations) which may reduce or amplify the risk. Taylor (2024) summarises how different reasons for offending can only be gleaned by determining the details of the event (what happened/why); cognitions (what was the offender thinking); emotional arousal (how did they react/why); and behaviours (what was done). For example, violence may stem from faulty cognitions

Table 14.1 Risk Assessment: Taking Students on a Court Visit.

Activity	Potential harm	Level of harm	Likelihood	Mitigation
Coach travel	Crash	Potentially high	Low	- Use reputable company - Wear seatbelts
Sitting in public gallery	Emotional distress	Potentially high	Medium	- Consider content in advance - Give briefing/ debrief - Provide aftercare/ support
	Abuse from others	Medium	Low	- Consider likely attendees e.g., ask court usher - Have a supervisor in each court room - Stay together

(e.g., perceiving hostile intent – 'he spilled his drink over me on purpose') leading to emotional arousal (anger) resulting in an inappropriate behavioural response (physical violence).

Conducting a risk assessment therefore "*involves many complex challenges*" (Crighton, 2023, p. 2) and as such, guidance is provided as to how risk can be measured.

Measurement of Risk

Measurement has historically focussed upon predicting the likelihood of **recidivism**.
Features such as the likelihood (is it likely to happen), severity (how serious will it be), frequency (how often) or imminence (how soon) of criminal behaviour taking place are considered. More recently, consideration of current individual needs (what offenders require) and level of risk posed (how 'dangerous' they currently are) have taken precedence (McGuire & Duff, 2018).

Recidivism. Reoffending.

Risk posed by offenders after sentencing was traditionally ('first generation' assessments) based on clinical judgement which was reached after reading case files and conducting interviews; risk was based on a clinician's knowledge/experience. Such opinions were criticised for subjectivity and as an understanding of risk factors developed, 'second generation' assessments including standardised actuarial, statistical measurements of risk were introduced. Practitioners could measure the risk of potential criminality based on **static factors** i.e., fixed and unchangeable (e.g., previous convictions, age) to predict future behaviour (Lewis, 2014). However, the importance of incorporating **dynamic risk factors** i.e., features which can be influenced or changed (e.g., being in a stable relationship, employment, attitudes) are now recognised (e.g., Yukhnenko et al., 2020).

Static Factors. Factors which cannot be changed (e.g., previous convictions).

Dynamic Factors. Factors which can be changed (e.g., employment).

Risk Factors. Increase the likelihood of a negative outcome (e.g., re-offending).

Protective Factors. Factors which help prevent reoffending (e.g., having positive role models).

Subsequently 'third generation' 'structured professional judgements' (SPJ) consider **risk factors** which increase the likelihood of re-offending and **protective factors** which protect against some of these, which can be both 'static' or 'dynamic'. The SPJ involve the use of empirically based checklists and guides, with the addition of professional expertise based on evidence from observations, interviews and case files; or theory, research and statistics (see Crighton, 2023 for a review). Importantly, these can be used to formulate a holistic understanding of the individual, flexibly estimating a likelihood of risk, while additionally considering potential treatment and future management plans.

Such tools have been criticised in relation to limited accuracy and sometimes poor predictive validity (e.g., Fazel, 2019). One systematic review, while acknowledging them as a good starting point, highlighted inconsistency in use by practitioners, with offender needs remaining unmet, labelling them mere 'bureaucratic exercises' (Viljoen et al., 2018).

'Fourth generation' assessments have been developed by the Ministry of Justice in the UK – **Offender Assessment Systems** (OASys), which incorporate both actuarial (statistical) and professional (clinical) judgement to consider the likelihood of reoffending. They include

> **Offender Assessment Systems.** Incorporate actuarial (statistical) and professional (clinical) judgement to consider the likelihood of reoffending and provide future management plans.

a broader range of factors for consideration in treatment (e.g., attitudes, health, employment, emotional wellbeing) ensuring assessment not only considers the likelihood of reconviction, but also provides clear, continual management plans – for example working more closely with probation post release. However, while focussing on risk and appropriate treatment, they do not require an underlying formulation to understand the reasoning behind offending behaviour.

A summary of the development of risk assessments over time, together with examples are provided in Table 14.2. However:

> *There are a wide range of valid criticisms of current forensic practice in the area of risk.*
>
> (Crighton, 2023, p. 2)

There are criticisms of statistical measures. A systematic review of data from 50 studies looking at 36 tools aimed to assess violence risk in forensic mental health from 12 countries. The review found mixed evidence of predictive performance and a high risk of bias calling for a review of practice (Ogonah et al., 2023). There are concerns regarding the subjectivity of professional judgements, even if structured, and some state the focus on risk assessment highlights the *deficits* of behaviour rather than the *strengths* of the whole person minimising consideration of individual differences which could be utilised to encourage desistance (e.g., Ward &

Table 14.2 Development of Risk Assessments.

Generation	Pros/cons	Example
1st Clinical Judgement 2nd Actuarial/Statistical	Susceptible to subjectivity • Can predict • Standardised • May not allow for bi-directional change • Limited consideration of context • Little application for treatment	One-to-one clinical interview Violence Risk Appraisal Guide (Harris, Rice & Quinsey, 1993). 12 items which • increase (e.g., violent criminal history) or • decrease (e.g., living with parents until age 16) prediction and likelihood of future violence
3rd Structured Professional Judgement	• More flexible • Greater inclusion of dynamic factors • Incorporates offender needs • Clear suggestions for treatment/management	HCR-20 (V3) (Douglas & Belfrage, 2015) – to establish risk of violence 20 risk factors under subscales • historical (e.g., response to treatment) • clinical (e.g., recent violent intent) • risk management: (e.g., future problems with stress/coping) Considers what factors lead to and maintain offending behaviour (e.g., situational triggers)
4th Systematic intervention and monitoring (developed by the Ministry of Justice)	• Broader range of risk factors • Enhances individuality of assessments • Allows for unified, on-going assessment and management • No formulation required	OASys prison and probation tool to identify • why individuals offend • what can help them desist Includes • different risk assessments • interview • self-assessment • acute risk factors (things that can change quickly)

Brown, 2004). Others highlight uncompromising statistics – for example figures published by the the Ministry of Justice in 2022 revealed that 59 offenders committed murder while either on probation or having recently left supervision (Gregory, 2023).

As such, balancing punishment and rehabilitation can be a difficult task. Moreover, attempts to maintain an individual's right to freedom whilst also protecting society can prove to be challenging and subject to controversy, as outlined in Box 14.1.

Box 14.1   Case study: Psychological assessments of John Worboys.

John Worboys (the 'Black Cab Rapist') was a serial sex offender – convicted of attacks on 16 women by drugging them in his taxi, then raping or sexually assaulting them.

After his arrest he was subject to many psychological assessments. Initially he maintained his innocence, but by 2015 he admitted responsibility and wished to discuss his offending. His motivation appeared genuine, and he was recommended for, and completed the Sex Offender Treatment Programme in 2016. Structured professional judgement assessment identified the need for more treatment, noting that if he continued to progress he may be ready to move to a lower category (security) prison.

In 2017 a request to move to an open prison was denied, however assessment from the Risk of Sexual Violence Protocol (SPJ) determined him low risk owing to his openness regarding his offending. A subsequent report highlighted his understanding of victim empathy and noted his remorse and shame – highlighting personal difficulties in the form of a break-up prior to offending. He was therefore considered a low risk (of sexual offending) and it was felt he could safely be managed in an open prison or if released. As such, later in 2017 the parole board approved his release.

However, new prosecutions were brought (resulting in subsequent convictions in 2019) and in 2018 the decision to release him was quashed. Despite appeals he still remains in prison.

http://news.bbc.co.uk/1/hi/england/london/7921
926.stm
www.judiciary.uk/wp-content/uploads/2019/12/Radf
ord-Sentence_.pdf
www.bbc.co.uk/news/uk-england-london-42571219
www.bbc.co.uk/news/uk-43568533
www.theguardian.com/uk-news/2021/feb/24/john-
worboys-rapist-loses-appeal-against-life-sentence

Risk Management

Once risks have been identified, and levels measured – consideration turns to how risks can be managed. Locking up all offenders indefinitely (see indeterminate sentences in further reading below) is impractical and ethically questionable, so interventions aim to reduce and manage the risk posed. For example, if someone is deemed 'high risk' of displaying violent behaviour when drinking alcohol, treatment interventions can be put in place to manage alcohol use, control anger, and teach alternative ways of resolving conflict.

The importance of risk management, and appropriate treatment is highlighted in Box 14.2, but is discussed further in Chapter 15.

Box 14.2   Case study: Risk management – Valdo Calocane.

On 13 June 2023 school caretaker Ian Coates (65 years) and students Barnaby Webber and Grace O'Malley-Kumar (both 19 years) were stabbed to death in Nottingham, UK.

The individual responsible, Valdo Calocane, suffered from paranoid delusions. Three years prior he was diagnosed with paranoid schizophrenia, but essential opportunities in his care had been missed via a *"series of errors, omissions and misjudgements"* and *"inconsistent approaches to risk assessment"* (Care Quality Commission, 2024). Parents of the deceased issued statements: *"looking at the management, treatment and delivery of care to Valdo Calocane is particularly*

> *disturbing, the treatment was completely inconsistent, it was inadequate, and it basically led to what happened on 13th June. This was a person with escalating violent behaviour, non-adherence to his medication and lack of engagement with his healthcare, so these are all risk factors for homicide,"* Dr Sinead O'Malley (mother of Grace O'Malley-Kumar, BBC News, 13/08/2024).
> www.bbc.co.uk/news/articles/cn47mm7ggv0o
> www.cqc.org.uk/publications/nottinghamshire-healthc are-nhsft-special-review-part2/summary

While such individuals may not be 'cured', with appropriate psychological interventions, therapeutic support, and access to resources, risks can be significantly mitigated (Parisi et al., 2021).

Summary

This chapter considered the importance of assessment in forensic domains focussing on the risk of re-offending. One way in which risks can be mitigated is in attempts to change offending behaviour via appropriate treatment – the subject of the following chapter.

Note

1 There are several potential outcomes of assessment of risk – the assessment of risk is correct or 'true' (e.g., the person is assessed as high risk and is high risk) or the assessment of risk is incorrect or 'false' – they may either have been deemed high risk and are not (false positive) or are high risk and have not been assessed as so (false negative). Obviously, the aim is to obtain as many 'true' and as few 'false' instances as possible.

Further Reading

Video – A series outlining decision making of Parole Boards can be seen here www.bbc.co.uk/iplayer/episodes/m001jfsn/parole

Web pages – Details of standards, and a list of users included on the Register of Qualifications in Test Use (RQTU) is here www.bps.org. uk/about-psychological-testing-centre

Sentencing guidelines assist judges in England and Wales when deciding the type and length of sentence to pass –www.sentencingcouncil.org. uk/sentencing-and-the-council/about-sentencing-guidelines/

Passing indeterminate sentences (with no set end date) in England and Wales has now ceased – however the interested reader is referred to https://prisonreformtrust.org.uk/adviceguide/understanding-your-sentence/#:~:text=An%20indeterminate%20sentence%20is%20a,is%20 called%20your%20%27tariff%27.

Podcasts– "The Forensic Psychology Podcast" has an episode discussing Risk Assessment with leading researchers in the field.

References

Brown, J., Shell, Y., & Cole, T. (2015). *Forensic psychology: Theory, research, policy and practice*. Sage.

Crighton, D. (2023). *Risk assessment in forensic practice*. Routledge.

Douglas, K. S., & Belfrage, H. (2015). The structured professional judgment approach to violence risk assessment and management. In C. A. Pietz & C. A. Mattson (Eds.), *Violent offenders: Understanding and assessment* (pp. 360–383). Oxford University Press.

Fazel, S. (2019). The scientific validity of current approaches to violence and criminal risk assessment. Predictive sentencing: normative and empirical perspectives. In J. W. de Keijser, J. V. Roberts, & J. Ryberg (Eds.), *Predictive sentencing. Normative and empirical perspective* (pp. 197–212). Hart Publishing. https://doi.org/10.5040/978150 9921447.ch-011

Gregory, A. (2023) *Criminals released from prison could be left free to kill as overstretched probation service in crisis*. The Independent. 13/11/ 2023.

Harris, G. T., Rice, M. E., & Quinsey, V. L. (1993). Violent recidivism of mentally disordered offenders: The development of a statistical prediction instrument. *Criminal Justice and Behavior*, *20*(4), 315–335.

Lewis, D. M. (2014). The risk factor – (Re-) visiting adult offender risk assessments within criminal justice practice. *Risk Management, 16*, 121–136. https://doi.org/10.1057/rm.2014.6

McGuire, J., & Duff, S. (2018). *Forensic psychology: Routes through the system*. Bloomsbury Publishing.

Ogonah, M. G., Seyedsalehi, A., Whiting, D., & Fazel, S. (2023). Violence risk assessment instruments in forensic psychiatric populations: A systematic review and meta-analysis. *The Lancet Psychiatry*, *10*(10), 780–789.

Parisi, A., Wilson, A. B., Villodas, M., Phillips, J., & Dohler, E. (2022). A systematic review of interventions targeting criminogenic risk factors among persons with serious mental illness. *Psychiatric Services, 73*(8), 897–909. https://doi.org/10.1176/appi.ps.202000928

Taylor, S. (2024). *Forensic psychology: The basics.* Routledge.

Viljoen, J. L., Cochrane, D. M., & Jonnson, M. R. (2018). Do risk assessment tools help manage and reduce risk of violence and reoffending? A systematic review. *Law and Human Behavior, 42*(3), 181. https://doi.org/10.1037/lhb0000280

Ward, T., & Brown, M. (2004). The good lives model and conceptual issues in offender rehabilitation. *Psychology, Crime & Law, 10*(3), 243–257.

Yukhnenko, D., Blackwood, N., & Fazel, S. (2020). Risk factors for recidivism in individuals receiving community sentences: a systematic review and meta-analysis. *CNS Spectrums, 25*(2), 252–263. https://doi.org/10.1017/S1092852919001056

Chapter 15

Treatment of Offenders

Key Points

Treatment of offenders involves attempts at rehabilitation or management to help reduce future offending.

Interventions can be general (e.g., teaching social skills) or specifically tailored for certain groups (e.g., violent offenders).

Cognitive behavioural therapies are common, focussing on behaviour change to reduce recidivism.

Consideration of individual needs and how to assist offenders build better lives is increasingly recognised.

What is Offender Treatment?

When we think of **treatment** we perhaps consider medical care given to a patient – to 'treat' an illness or condition, make it better, or reduce the likelihood of pain. In a forensic domain in order to **manage** offenders to reduce (or ideally cease) future offending, some form of treatment may be required.

Treatment Of Offenders. Approaches used to help offenders change behaviours and attitudes which may facilitate criminal behaviour.

Management of Offenders. Managing time/supervision of offenders (usually aiming to reduce reoffending).

DOI: 10.4324/9781003431213-19

As seen in the previous chapter, assessments are made to determine whether offenders are ready for, and what kind of treatment may be of benefit. Treatments may be tailored to offending behaviour (e.g., sex offences), specific problems (e.g., substance abuse) or bespoke needs (e.g., managing anger). They can take many forms (e.g., group work), may only be offered in certain environments (e.g., while in prison), with caveats (e.g., cannot concurrently engage in substance misuse) and to specific groups (e.g., offenders deemed high risk of reoffending).

When is Management and Treatment Applicable?

Management of unwanted behaviour can occur at any time, including prior to offending. Individuals themselves, or others may recognise inappropriate behaviour, and steps may be taken to manage this. For example, a relationship may display elements of control (checking a partner's phone or suggesting they stay at home rather than go out with friends), which may initially be managed by conversation ('why do you want to see my phone?') and/or action (seeing friends one night, partner another). However, when behaviours become harmful (e.g., the phone is grabbed; or someone repeatedly reacts badly when their partner goes out) then further steps may be required. Those who display such behaviours in domestic situations, may proactively engage in treatment to assist them for example.

Often however, management and treatment occur after an offence has been committed. Interventions to reduce or at least manage the risk posed by individuals may be mandated by an agency or court (conditions as part of a sentence) or may be undertaken voluntarily in the community.

Who Can be Treated?

Ideally anyone who is engaging in unwanted or criminal behaviour should have access to treatment. However, there are many reasons why people may not engage. In relation to domestic abuse, barriers to seeking treatment can include embarrassment/shame, or help may not be readily available (see Harvey et al., 2024). A lack of funding, location (courses may be some distance away), or eligibility issues may also hinder access.

Zara et al. (2020) also summarise challenges to 'treatment readiness' including the offender's motivation to change (they may not want to); denial (saying they are innocent or thinking they have not done anything wrong) and/or minimisation (recounting things differently – minimising their level involvement). Moreover, particular populations may be difficult to treat – such as psychopathic offenders.

Interventions

Typically, offending behaviour can be managed by custodial confinement, supervision by staff, medical or psychological **interventions**, and, particularly in the community – support from professionals, peers/family. Interventions can be general (e.g., teaching social skills) or specific for different groups (e.g., anger management for violent offenders). They can be provided in a variety of ways – one to one or in a group, using a range of approaches. In terms of sex offending, Lösel and Schmucker (2017) highlight diverse methods used including cognitive-behavioural courses (see below), **relapse prevention programmes, psychodynamic counselling**, being housed in **therapeutic communities** (see Shuker & Shine, 2010; Warren, 2010), and even **surgical castration** has been used (see Diaz, 2024).

Interventions. Actions taken to help change behaviour or feelings (e.g., offender treatment).

Relapse Prevention Programmes. Identify and manage situations which increase the risk of offending to 'prevent relapse'.

Psychodynamic Counselling. Considers how unconscious processes may affect behaviour.

Therapeutic Communities. Units/institutions where people live and learn together via access to programmes, treatments, and activities. Democratically run by the users/offenders with staff.

Surgical Castration. Removal of testicles or ovaries to stop production of sex hormones.

Table 15.1 Risk-Need-Responsivity.

R-N-R	Targets	Action
Risk	Who to treat	Provide treatment proportional to the offender's level of risk
Need	What to treat	Focus on criminogenic needs
Responsivity	How to treat	Matching the offender's abilities, motivation, learning style to treatment delivery

In terms of treatment to reduce recidivism, many interventions are based on the **Risk-Need-Responsivity** (R-N-R) Principles (Bonta & Andrews, 2007) summarised in Table 15.1.

Such approaches often utilise **Cognitive Behavioural Therapy (CBT)** which has been used worldwide. This considers how people think (cognitive) and act (behavioural) in particular situations, aiming to change dysfunctional

Risk-Need-Responsivity. Treatment provided based on levels of risk, focussing on criminogenic needs and delivered responsively considering offender abilities and needs.

Criminogenic Needs. Factors related to offending behaviour (e.g., having antisocial associates).

Cognitive Behavioural Therapy (CBT). Helps manage problems/offending by changing the way individuals think and behave.

attitudes and maladaptive thoughts (Smith et al., 2024). Mainly group-based programmes include teaching skills to motivate offenders in setting goals and making realistic plans to reduce reoffending. Methods are standardised, with explicit manuals providing detail of course structure and delivery. A variety of programmes include topics reflecting reasoning, aggression, and relationships.

In response to criticisms regarding the narrow (and demotivating) focus on offence behaviour; and measuring success predominantly in terms of desistance; increasingly interventions consider more holistic rehabilitation. Proponents of the **Good Lives Model** (GLM, e.g. Ward & Stewart, 2003) propose working and engaging with (rather than 'doing to') the 'whole' person (only *part* of whom is an 'offender'), considering their strengths as well as their weaknesses, which enhances and promotes a prosocial lifestyle. This approach is flexible, considering the variety of motivations for committing and maintaining offending. For example, once offenders are released from prison they may reoffend owing to being subjected to the same (or enhanced) life challenges they had before (e.g., criminal associations, lack of skills). Consideration of what an offender wants (e.g., money) and collaboratively identifying how they can get there (e.g., training) to obtain their ultimate goals (e.g., a fulfilling job, home, family) provides individualised support. It also has a broader emphasis rather than focussing only on criminality, providing more comprehensive measurements of success than desistance alone. In turn, working together and endorsing acceptance of personal responsibility are more likely to lead to maintenance of an offence free lifestyle. The GLM has been adopted in many countries including USA, Canada and Australasia (see Zeccola et al., 2021), and the current Prison Strategy in the UK (Ministry of Justice, 2021, 2022) recognises that offenders should leave prison with a 'firm foundation' of employment opportunities, assistance with mental health and substance abuse issues, and stronger family ties, by services working collaboratively and with offenders.

> **Good Lives Model (GLM).** Approach to offender rehabilitation focussing on building strengths together with an individual to assist them in living a good, prosocial, offending free future life.

In the UK, a full list of programmes accredited for use in prison or the community are published by the Correctional Service Advice and Accreditation Panel who review products (Ministry of Justice, 2023). Programmes include alcohol dependence, building better relationships, controlling anger or violence, and those focussing on specific offence types such as serious sex offending. All developed in order to address maladaptive behaviours.

Box 15.1   Case study: Use of Schema Therapy with a convicted murderer.

The use of schema therapy assisted a male convicted of raping and murdering his wife by processing his previous experiences of neglect (from his foster parents) and trauma (from his own sexual abuse victimisation), and subsequently enabling him to develop meaningful relationships to meet his emotional needs (Yapp, 2019).

The offender was caught in repeating patterns using emotional detachment or giving in to others' demands to protect himself from hurt. Sometimes when these coping methods did not work or if he felt threatened, he overcompensated resulting in aggression or violence. As such he had difficulties building and maintaining secure relationships.

By using role play, keeping diaries, and educating him to monitor and be aware of the links between his previous experiences and current behavioural responses, he succeeded in identifying and changing his behaviour – for example socialising more with peers on the ward – enhancing his personal relationships; and modifying his responses – replacing his prior violent reactions with alternative means of coping.

Accessible examples of case studies detailing how assessments and treatments are undertaken by forensic psychologists are provided by Tully and Bamford (2019). One is outlined in Box 15.1. **Schema therapy** helps clients identify and break long-standing, problematic self-defeating patterns of negative feelings and beliefs (e.g., 'people will leave me'), and develop healthier alternatives to replace them (see Young, 1999).

Schema Therapy. Helps clients identify and break patterns of negative feelings and beliefs and develop healthier alternatives.

Does it Work (and How Can We Find Out)?

There are difficulties in measuring success of treatment. Using the example of sex offender treatment, Zara et al. (2020) highlight that some individuals may not have access to treatment, some do not accept it, some are excluded (e.g., owing to complete denial), or drop out part way through.

In addition, attributing change directly to the treatment or intervention can be problematic. At the end of group treatment some participants may desist while others may go on to offend, therefore 'success' in terms of recidivism may be mixed. Moreover, those who desist may do so because of the treatment received or they may have ceased or 'grown out' of offending anyway, for example if they ceased to associate with criminal peers. Also, there are debates regarding how long individuals should be tracked to see if they have re-offended – owing to timescales of much funded research, follow-ups tend to be short term. In addition, if someone stops committing serious crime, but still commits lesser offences – is this success? Or if they were stealing twice a day and now shoplift twice a year is this improvement? Many crimes are not reported, may not be recorded and many are unsolved – as such a lack of a subsequent criminal record, may not equate to a lack of subsequent offending. As there are so many influential variables, even reoffending measurement is difficult.

Initial suggestions highlighted that very little was shown to 'work' in terms of treatment and rehabilitation of offenders:

These data, involving over two hundred studies and hundreds of thousands of individuals ... give us very little reason to hope that we have in fact found a sure way of reducing recidivism through rehabilitation. This is not to say that we found no instances of success or partial success; it is only to say that these instances have been isolated, producing no clear pattern to indicate the efficacy of any particular method of treatment.

Martinson, 1974, p. 49.

However, nearly 50 years later:

The effect of interventions depends on both the quality of treatment ... the individual's responses to treatment and motivation to change ... any change is likely to be linked to deliberate interventions (e.g., rehabilitation programmes).

Zara et al., 2020, p. 169.

Current evidence indicates that if people change, this is likely to be linked to interventions, but this is inconsistent – some treatments work for some people some of the time. Cognitive-behavioural methods have been shown to be particularly effective (e.g., Hanson et al., 2002; Schmucker & Lösel, 2015) because of their focus on teaching offenders to reconsider attitudes and thoughts, think about implications and consequences of behaviours, and learn methods to control them. There has been much support for R-N-R programmes outlined above in terms of efficacy in reduction of future offending (e.g., Bonta & Andrews, 2016; Hanson et al., 2009), however the impact from GLM models remains mixed (Zeccola et al., 2021). Programmes with an individual (rather than all group based) element were found to be beneficial, as were programmes delivered to a high-quality standard (Schmucker & Lösel, 2015). However, debates continue as to whether such measures are sufficient, or whether broader considerations for a wider recovery – e.g., whether offenders go on to live happy, fulfilling lives integrated within society – should be the aim (see Laws & Ward, 2011). Yet measuring other features such as relatedness[1], inner peace[2] or pleasure[3] for example, may be even more problematic.

Summary

Despite a variety of treatment methods, debate continues as to 'what works' and how best to measure this. Ongoing assistance, self-reflection and reintegration may be pivotal in providing both a better life for the offender, and have better outcomes for society.

Notes

1 Positive relationships
2 Freedom from turmoil and stress
3 Feeling good presently

Further Reading

Websites – The UK Ministry of Justice, HM Prison and Probation Service publish details of offending behaviour programmes here www. gov.uk/guidance/offending-behaviour-programmes-and-interventi ons#:~:text=Offender%20behaviour%20programmes%20and%20interv entions,self-mangement

The Good Lives Model has a website: www.goodlivesmodel.com

Videos – An interesting documentary considering if sex offenders can change www.youtube.com/watch?v=KjjGJBoviHE

An offender describing how he turned his life around www.youtube.com/watch?v=PYgJN2aKspA

Podcasts – "The Forensic Psychology Podcast" has an episode called How do we help people change?

"More Than My Past" features interviews of offenders who have experienced rehabilitation and how approaches to crime can be improved.

References

Bonta, J., & Andrews, D. A. (2007). Risk-need-responsivity model for offender assessment and rehabilitation. *Rehabilitation*, *6*(1), 1–22.

Bonta, J., & Andrews, D. A. (2016). *The psychology of criminal conduct.* Routledge.

Diaz, J. (January 7, 2024) What to know about Louisiana's new surgical castration law. NPR News Retrieved January 28, 2025, from www. npr.org/2024/07/01/nx-s1-5020686/louisiana-new-surgical-castrat ion-law

Hanson, R. K., Bourgon, G., Helmus, L., & Hodgson, S. (2009). The principles of effective correctional treatment also apply to sexual offenders: A meta-analysis. *Criminal Justice and Behavior*, *36*(9), 865–891.

Hanson, R. K., Gordon, A., Harris, A. J., Marques, J. K., Murphy, W., Quinsey, V. L., & Seto, M. C. (2002). First report of the collaborative outcome data project on the effectiveness of psychological treatment for sex offenders. *Sexual Abuse: A Journal of Research and Treatment*, *14*, 169–194.

Harvey, O., Cole, T., Levell, J., & Healy, J. (2024). Explorations of attitudes towards accessibility and accessing domestic violence and abuse (DVA) perpetrator support programmes by victim-survivors and perpetrators across five European countries. *Abuse: An International Impact Journal*, *5*(1), 26–45.

Laws, D. R., & Ward, T. (2011). *Desistance from sex offending: Alternatives to throwing away the keys.* Guilford Press.

Lösel, F., & Schmucker, M. (2017). Treatment of sex offenders: Concepts and empirical evaluations. In T. Sanders (Ed.), *The Oxford handbook of sex offences and sex offenders* (pp. 392–414). Oxford University Press. doi: 10.1093/oxfordhb/9780190213633.013.23

Martinson, R. (1974). What works? Questions and answers about prison reform. *The Public Interest, 35*(2), 22–54.

Ministry of Justice. (2021). Prisons Strategy White Paper. Retrieved March 22, 2025, from https://assets.publishing.service.gov.uk/media/61af18e38fa8f5037e8ccc47/prisons-strategy-white-paper.pdf

Ministry of Justice. (2022). Prisons Strategy White Paper – Response to Consultation Questions. Retrieved March 22, 2025, from https://assets.publishing.service.gov.uk/media/62a71a37d3bf7f03744c7c4a/prisons-strategy-white-paper-govt-response.pdf

Ministry of Justice. (2023). HMPPS Accredited Programmes. Retrieved March 22, 2025, from https://view.officeapps.live.com/op/view.aspx?src=https%3A%2F%2Fassets.publishing.service.gov.uk%2Fmedia%2F64085767e90e0740d3cd6fa3%2FHMPPS_Accredited_Programmes.docx&wdOrigin=BROWSELINK

Schmucker, M., & Lösel, F. (2015). The effects of sexual offender treatment on recidivism: An international meta-analysis of sound quality evaluations. *Journal of Experimental Criminology, 11*, 597–630.

Shuker, R., & Shine, J. (2010). The role of therapeutic communities in forensic settings: developments, research, and adaptations. In J. Harvey & K. Smedley (Eds.), *Psychological therapy in prisons and other settings* (pp. 215–230). Willan Publishing

Smith, A., Roberts, A., Krzemieniewska-Nandwani, K., Eggins, E., Cook, W., Fox, C., & Szifris, K. (2024). Revisiting the effectiveness of cognitive-behavioural therapy for reducing reoffending in the criminal justice system: A systematic review. *Campbell Systematic Reviews, 20*(3), e1425.

Tully, R., & Bamford, J. (Eds.). (2019). *Case studies in forensic psychology: Clinical assessment and treatment.* Routledge.

Ward, T., & Stewart, C. A. (2003). The treatment of sex offenders: Risk management and good lives. *Professional Psychology: Research and Practice, 34*(4), 353–360. https://doi.org/10.1037/0735-7028.34.4.353

Warren, F. (2010). Therapeutic communities. In J. M., Brown & E. Campbell (Eds.), *The Cambridge handbook of forensic psychology.* Cambridge University Press.

Yapp, J. (2019). Male personality disorder: Treatment approaches within a secure mental health setting. In R. Tully & J. Bamford (Eds.), *Case studies in forensic psychology* (pp. 48–69). Routledge.

Young, J. E. (1999). *Cognitive therapy for personality disorders: A schema-focused approach.* Professional Resource Press/Professional Resource Exchange.

Zara, G., Farrington, D. P., Freilone, F., & Lösel, F. (2020). Assessment, management, and treatment of sex offenders: What is known, what is controversial, what needs further investigation. *Rassegna Italiana di Criminologia, 3,* 166–185.

Zeccola, J., Kelty, S. F., & Boer, D. (2021). Does the good lives model work? A systematic review of the recidivism evidence. *The Journal of Forensic Practice, 23*(3), 285–300.

Part V

Key Emerging Areas

Chapter 16

Where Do We Go from Here

Future Research

Key Points

Research drives reliable and valid application of psychology in practice.
 Research needs to account for changes in societal and practitioner needs.
 A mix of research methods are required and can utilise new technologies.

The Need for Research

As highlighted throughout this book research is the backbone driving the application of forensic and investigative psychology approaches and

Research. Systematic inquiry involving collecting, evaluating and analysing data to enhance understanding/knowledge.

embedding them in practice. From the laboratory to the prison, court or incident room, much good practice has been cited. An example of this is the work of Charlie Frowd in relation to EvoFIT described in Box 16.1.

DOI: 10.4324/9781003431213-21

Box 16.1   Applications in real life: EvoFIT.

Witnesses and victims of crime are often asked to provide descriptions of offenders and where possible, provide a sketch of what the offender looked like. Traditionally these were done via drawings, then as computer software developed Photofit, identikit and e-fits of suspects were introduced. Witnesses could 'choose' individual facial features adding different types of hairstyle, glasses, etc. to their composite. However, these were largely ineffective in identifying suspects.

One example of how research developed from the laboratory in 1998, was piloted in practice, amended and re-tested, and is now used in police forces internationally – is EvoFIT. Rather than piecing 'parts' of a face together, this method looks at the whole face, focussing on the (most identifiable) central region around the eyes. It works by creating a set of faces with random facial features then getting users to select those that most resemble the suspect. These are combined, to develop a final composite of acceptable likeness. Therefore, it does not require the potentially less reliable *recall* of the details of an offender's face – merely *recognition* of suggested faces. The tool has enhanced suspect identification ten times greater than traditional methods (with over 70% correct identification).

See Erickson et al., 2024; Frowd, 2001; Frowd et al., 2010, 2011, 2019.

Such research is necessary, however obtaining funding for research can be difficult, particularly for longitudinal studies or follow ups. Monies for research are available via funding streams (see further reading) but can be competitive. Thankfully academia has moved away from prioritising excellence merely via publication of research papers in academic journals (often unread by practitioners – Lum et al., 2012). Increasingly research is expanding and researchers are considering the **impact** it has outside academia to wider society (see further reading) and realising the value of engaging with practitioners and responding to topics they require answers on.

Impact (research). Effect of research outside of academia.

Simultaneously, there is a greater demand from practitioners – who have recognised the need for research to assist them in resolving problems. Increasingly practitioners are held accountable for actions (be it locally via management, or nationally from public inquiries), and research can provide an underlying evidence base for decisions made.

Increasing professionalisation and recognition of the need for diversity has been enhanced by broader recruitment into professional roles. For example, in the UK the national policing Uplift programme enabled the recruitment of 20,000 additional police officers to enhance capacity and diversity, and there are now a broader variety of roles and routes into policing and other criminal justice careers (see further reading). Many roles now require further study, and **continual professional development** which often requires engagement with additional training, study or research. Rather than being a 'practitioner/

Continual Professional Development. Continual learning for professionals to maintain/enhance competence.

academic' divide, practitioners (like the first author) increasingly undertake further study and move from practice to working in academia, or vice versa. In addition, practitioners and academics working together on joint research projects is increasingly commonplace.

Future Topics

This joint working has led to a proliferation of new and interesting areas of research driven by social need, and of applied use to practitioners. While research on offenders still dominates the literature, and focussing on victim experiences is still less prevalent, journal publications have broadened their initial narrow focus from witness testimony to many different areas of interest (Brown et al., 2022). Rather than academics second guessing areas of need (or worse merely researching areas of interest to them), topics are increasingly focussed on areas of political and societal importance. An example has been the expanding focus on violence and women and girls (VAWG), leading to Operation Bluestone Soteria (see further reading). This is likely to stay top of the political agenda and as such further research will continue, enhancing what is known, and addressing how we can practically address abuse of all kinds (e.g., stalking, domestic abuse, non-fatal strangulation, coercive control, honour-based abuse). Other recent examples include consideration of **chemsex** (Jaspal, 2022); domestic violence and abuse in LGBTQIA[1]+, people with disabilities and BME[2] communities (Cole et al., 2025 – see Chapter 9), missing persons (Phoenix & Francis, 2023) and **female genital mutilation** (El-Dirani et al., 2022). As seen in Chapters 14 and 15 types of assessment and treatment are also continually under review and improvements are ongoing.

Chemsex. Sex under the influence of drugs, mostly among men who have sex with men.
Female Genital Mutilation. Cutting, changing or damaging female genitals.

Another example is work in relation to abuse of position in the police for sexual gain (see Sweeting et al., 2022; Sweeting & Cole, 2023a, 2023b) driven by significant cases such as the murder of Sarah Everard in the UK (see further reading), and the recognition of the increasing number of cases of people in authority abusing their positions. This has been researched in public figures (e.g., Scott, 2016), entertainment (e.g., Department of Health and Social Care, 2014), sport (e.g., Hartill, 2013; Timon et al., 2022), business (e.g., Erooga et al., 2020), education (Canning, 2022), and the medical profession (e.g., Mulvihill, 2022).

The increasing worldwide threat from **cybercrime** (Kuzior et al., 2024) has also led to research. Specific texts combine **cyberpsychology** and forensic psychology to look at psychological factors influencing behaviours (McAlaney et al., 2024) and examples of other research activities are **phishing** and online identity theft (Steele & McManus, 2023), and **romance scams** (Bilz et al., 2023).

Cybercrime. Criminal activities using computers/internet.

Cyberpsychology. How individuals interact/are affected by technology.

Phishing. Tricking others to give away sensitive information (e.g., sending scam emails).

Romance Scams. Feigning romantic interest to steal money.

While the variation in prevalence statistics for **human trafficking** is recognised (e.g., Van Dijk, 2024), human trafficking is known to harm millions worldwide, calling for a greater understanding (e.g., Barrick & Pfeffer, 2024; Steele & McManus, 2023). Increasingly research is being undertaken regarding **modern slavery** (e.g., Han et al., 2024) and working groups involving academics and practitioners are collaborating to deal with current knowledge and research gaps (e.g., the Human Trafficking Research Network[3]).

Human Trafficking. Involuntary movement for exploitation.

Modern Slavery. Exploitation by others for personal/commercial gain – e.g., human trafficking, forced labour, domestic servitude, slavery.

Terrorism. Use of threat to advance political, religious, racial or ideological aims to influence government or intimidate the public.

Radicalisation. Adopting extreme views which can lead to violence.

Recognition of global crimes such as **terrorism** and **radicalisation** has led to research groups considering security threats (see further reading). For instance, the rise of right-wing **extremism** and its potential impact on society (e.g.,

Extremism. Extreme ideology or views.

Gaudette et al., 2022) – is exemplified in the violent disorder the UK witnessed in the summer of 2024 through clashes between anti-immigration and Stand Up to Racism demonstrators; and seen more recently in anti-extremism protests early 2025 in Germany.

Future Methods

In the above-mentioned research, Gaudette et al. (2022) used interviews with former right-wing extremists to understand their use of the Internet, and the interplay between their online and off-line worlds. This is an example of utilising the 'voice of' participants in research – listening and advocating the voices of victims, witnesses, children, offenders and practitioners – realising that those with **lived experience** have untapped practical knowledge of topics

Lived Experience. Knowledge from personal experiences.

and can often suggest potential solutions. This can in part overcome sampling issues concerning only researching victims/survivors/offenders who are already within the criminal justice system, as it can include experiences of those involved in unreported incidents or undetected crimes. The importance of understanding different perspectives and impacts on all involved in criminal justice is being increasingly recognised (for an interesting account of the different parties impacted by rape see Brown et al., 2023).

Moreover, asking practitioners for their problems, and working together in an attempt to provide potential suggestions and solutions is the remit of **pragmatic psychology** (see Butt, 2013; Fishman, 1999). This turns the tables on the academics being the only experts or being

Pragmatic Psychology. Research focussing on practitioner problems, working together to provide solutions.

the only ones able to provide appropriate solutions – yet still ensures robust methods of research.

Yet while a recent **bibliometric review** of 3,719 journal articles published between 2015–2020 advocated the utility of qualitative research methods such as interviewing those involved, it identified

Bibliometric Review. Counting publications to map topics/methods.

that two thirds of forensic psychology research still focussed on quantitative methods (Brown et al., 2022). Despite some challenges in certain fields (see e.g., Turner et al., 2023), randomised control trials are still considered the gold standard (Brown et al., 2022; Duan et al., 2024; Ede et al., 2023). However, there has also been a call to utilise large datasets with 'big data' (see DeLisi, 2018) yet this may bring additional difficulties such as ethical considerations surrounding obtaining informed consent and retaining confidentiality.

Utilisation of newer forms of technology in research is also being undertaken. For example, researchers have explored the use of **virtual reality** to enhance the ecological validity of studies (Herman et al., 2024), and the use of innovative tools – such as analysis of social media comments (via forums such as https://nodexl.com) are now being incorporated. Recent collaborative research has utilised

Virtual Reality. Computer generated simulations to create immersive experience.

Artificial Intelligence. Computers/machines replicating human cognitive abilities.

Artificial Intelligence (AI) to highlight continual overuse of victim-blaming language by judges in family court (Hall, 2024); AI is also advocated as a method to speed up and improve accuracy of analysis – for example analysing reliability of testimonies (see Mavry et al., 2024).

Summary

This chapter provided examples of the broadening of topics and methods currently being utilised in forensic and investigative psychology research. Consideration beyond the criminal courts, into civil law and family courts, and broadening research into utilising samples beyond the Western world are sparse yet increasing. Topics and methods should develop in line with societal change and importantly be applied into developing practice – the topic of our final chapter.

Notes

1   Lesbian, Gay, Bisexual, Transgender, Queer, Intersex, Asexual
2   Black and Minority Ethnic
3   A Bournemouth University and National Chief Police Council collaboration.

Further Reading

Websites – Research/reports regarding topics discussed:

* Evofit – https://evofit.co.uk
* Operation Soteria/Bluestone – www.npcc.police.uk/our-work/violence-against-women-and-girls/operation-soteria
* Security threats – https://crestresearch.ac.uk
* Historical abuse of position reports into Jimmy Savile – www.gov.uk/government/collections/nhs-and-department-of-health-investigations-into-jimmy-savile

Funding streams:

* www.findaphd.com
* https://aafpforensic.org/grants/
* https://ampsychfdn.org/funding/
* www.ukri.org/councils/esrc/
* https://research-and-innovation.ec.europa.eu/funding/funding-opportunities/funding-programmes-and-open-calls/horizon-europe_en

The importance of 'impact' www.ukri.org/who-we-are/research-england/research-excellence/ref-impact
Videos – The UK police uplift programme www.youtube.com/watch?v=P3Wh5wTezJI
Police officers who abuse their position www.channel4.com/news/cops-on-trial-sexual-misconduct-and-the-police
An elite squad in Spain attempting to free trafficked women www.youtube.com/watch?v=nO2YU2DYi5g

References

Barrick, K., & Pfeffer, R. (2024). Advances in measurement: A scoping review of prior human trafficking prevalence studies and recommendations for future research. *Journal of Human Trafficking*, *10*(1), 1–19.

Bilz, A., Shepherd, L. A., & Johnson, G. I. (2023). Tainted love: A systematic literature review of online romance scam research. *Interacting with Computers*, *35*(6), 773–788.

Brown, J., Figueiredo, M., & Horvath, M. (2022) Taking stock; a review of the state of forensic psychology as revealed through an analysis of journal articles 2015-20. *Journal of Forensic Psychology Research and Practice*. *24*(2), 170–191. https://doi.org/10.1080/24732850.2022.2088326

Brown, J., Shell, Y., & Cole, T. (2023). *Revealing rape's many voices: Differing roles, reactions and reflections.* Palgrave Macmillan.

Butt, T. (2013). Toward a pragmatic psychology. *Journal of Constructivist Psychology*, *26*(3), 218–224.

Canning, D. L. (2022). Teachers who sexually abuse their students: A Systematic Review. Unpublished MRes Thesis. University of Huddersfield. https://pure.hud.ac.uk/ws/portalfiles/portal/67011906/FINAL_THESIS.pdf

Cole, T., Harvey, O., Healy, J. C., & Smith, C. (2025). Contemporary treatment of crime victims/survivors: Barriers faced by minority groups in accessing and utilizing domestic abuse services. *Behavioral Sciences*, *15*(2), 103.

DeLisi, M. (2018). The big data potential of epidemiological studies for criminology and forensics. *Journal of Forensic and Legal Medicine*, *57*, 24–27.

Department of Health and Social Care. (2014). *Investigations into Jimmy Savile.* www.gov.uk/government/collections/nhs-and-department-of-health-investigations-into-jimmy-savile

Duan, W., Wang, Z., Yang, C., & Ke, S. (2024). Are risk-need-responsivity principles golden? A meta-analysis of randomized controlled trials of community correction programs. *Journal of Experimental Criminology*, *20*(2), 593–616.

Ede, M. O., Okeke, C. I., & Onah, S. O. (2023). A randomised controlled trial of a cognitive behaviourally informed intervention for changing violent sexual attitudes among adult sexual offenders in prison. *Criminal Behaviour and Mental Health*, *33*(1), 46–61.

El-Dirani, Z., Farouki, L., Akl, C., Ali, U., Akik, C., & McCall, S. J. (2022). Factors associated with female genital mutilation: A systematic review and synthesis of national, regional and community-based studies. *BMJ Sexual & Reproductive Health*, *48*(3), 169–178.

Erickson, W. B., Brown, C., Portch, E., Lampinen, J. M., Marsh, J. E., Fodarella, C., ... & Frowd, C. D. (2024). The impact of weapons and unusual objects on the construction of facial composites. *Psychology, Crime & Law*, *30*(3), 207–228.

Erooga, M., Kaufman, K., & Zatkin, J. G. (2020). Powerful perpetrators, hidden in plain sight: An international analysis of organisational child sexual abuse cases. *Journal of Sexual Aggression*, *26*(1), 62–90.

Fishman, D. (1999). *The case for pragmatic psychology*. NYU Press.

Frowd, C. D. (2001). *EvoFIT: A holistic, evolutionary facial imaging system*. www.storre.stir.ac.uk/bitstream/1893/54/1/CharlieFrowd ThesisPlusCorrectionsDR.pdf

Frowd, C. D., Hancock, P. J., Bruce, V., McIntyre, A. H., Pitchford, M., Atkins, R., & Sendrea, G. (2010, September). Giving crime the'evo': Catching criminals using EvoFIT facial composites. In *2010 International Conference on Emerging Security Technologies* (pp. 36–43). IEEE.

Frowd, C. D., Hancock, P. J., Bruce, V., Skelton, F. C., Atherton, C. J., Nelson, L., ... & Sendrea, G. (2011). Catching more offenders with EvoFIT facial composites: Lab research and police field trials. *Global Journal of Human-Social Science*, *11*(3), 35–46.

Frowd, C. D., Portch, E., Killeen, A., Mullen, L., Martin, A. J., & Hancock, P. J. (2019, July). EvoFIT facial composite images: A detailed assessment of impact on forensic practitioners, police investigators, victims, witnesses, offenders and the media. In *2019 Eighth International Conference on Emerging Security Technologies (EST)* (pp. 1–7). IEEE.

Gaudette, T., Scrivens, R., & Venkatesh, V. (2022). The role of the internet in facilitating violent extremism: Insights from former right-wing extremists. *Terrorism and Political Violence*, *34*(7), 1339–1356.

Hall, R. (2024, October 8). Family court judges use victim blaming language in domestic abuse cases, finds AI project. Retrieved March 8, 2025, from www.theguardian.com/law/2024/oct/08/family-court-judges-victim-blaming-language-domestic-abuse-cases-ai-project

Han, C., Jia, F., Jiang, M., & Chen, L. (2024). Modern slavery in supply chains: A systematic literature review. *International Journal of Logistics Research and Applications*, *27*(7), 1206–1227.

Hartill, M. (2013). Concealment of child sexual abuse in sports. *Quest*, *65*(2), 241–254.

Herman, S., Barnum, T. C., Minà, P. E., Wozniak, P., & Van Gelder, J. L. (2024). Affect, emotions, and crime decision-making: Emerging insights from immersive 360 video experiments. *Journal of Experimental Criminology*, 1–34. https://doi.org/10.1007/s11292-024-09615-y

Jaspal, R. (2022). Chemsex, identity and sexual health among gay and bisexual men. *International Journal of Environmental Research and Public Health, 19*(19), 12124.

Kuzior, A., Tiutiunyk, I., Zielińska, A., & Kelemen, R. (2024). Cybersecurity and cybercrime: Current trends and threats. *Journal of International Studies (2071-8330), 17*(2). www.jois.eu/files/12_144 1_JIS_Tiutiunyk%20et%20al.pdf

Lum, C., Telep, C. W., Koper, C. S., & Grieco, J. (2012). Receptivity to research in policing. *Justice Research and Policy, 14*(1), 61–95.

McAlaney, J., Hills, P. J., & Cole, T. (2024). *Forensic perspectives on cyber-crime: Human behaviour and cybersecurity.* Taylor & Francis.

Mavry, B., Aseri, V., Nagar, V., Rai, A. R., Jain, D., Sharma, A., & Parihar, K. (2024). Emerging technology in criminal investigation systems. In K. Saini, S. S. Sonone, M. S. Sankhla, N. Kumar (Eds.), *Artificial intelligence in forensic psychology* (pp. 130–141). CRC Press.

Mulvihill, N. (2022). Professional authority and sexual coercion: A paradigmatic case study of doctor abuse. *Social Science & Medicine, 305,* 115093.

Phoenix, J., & Francis, B. J. (2023). Police risk assessment and case outcomes in missing person investigations. *The Police Journal, 96*(3), 390–410.

Scott, E. (2016). Historical child sexual abuse investigations. House of Lords Library Note. https://researchbriefings.files.parliament.uk/documents/LLN-2016-0033/LLN-2016-0033.pdf

Steele, R., & McManus, M. (2023). Forensic psychology and future directions. In K. Corteen, R. Steel, N. Cross & M. McManus (Eds.), *Forensic psychology, crime and policing* (pp. 83–88). Policy Press.

Sweeting, F., Cole, T., & Hills, P. (2022). Is the blue wall of silence a fallacy in cases of police sexual misconduct? *International Journal of Police Science & Management, 24*(3), 285–297.

Sweeting, F., & Cole, T. (2023a). Sexual misconduct in police recruits as identified by police trainers. *The Police Journal, 96*(2), 245–266.

Sweeting, F., & Cole, T. (2023b). The sharks and the fishermen: An exploratory content analysis of police officers who abused their positions for a sexual purpose. *International Journal of Police Science & Management, 25*(4), 368–378.

Timon, C. E., Dallam, S. J., Hamilton, M. A., Liu, E., Kang, J. S., Ortiz, A. J., & Gelles, R. J. (2022). Child sexual abuse of elite athletes: Prevalence, perceptions, and mental health. *Journal of Child Sexual Abuse, 31*(6), 672–691.

Turner, W., Morgan, K., Hester, M., Feder, G., & Cramer, H. (2023). Methodological challenges in group-based randomised controlled trials for intimate partner violence perpetrators: A meta-summary. *Psychosocial Intervention*, *32*(2), 123.

Van Dijk, J. (2024). Making statistics on human trafficking work. *Journal of Human Trafficking*, *10*(2), 339–345.

Chapter 17

Where Do We Go from Here

Future Practice

Key Points

Evidence-based practice incorporates research findings into practice.
  Policy and practice should:

- consider the voices of those involved in the criminal justice system
- develop alongside changes in criminality and society

  Supervision, reflective practice and peer review are advocated.

Evidence-based practice (EBP) is the incorporation of findings from (usually research) evidence, into practice. For example, if we know a treatment reduced reoffending in 99% of cases, practice would be enhanced by offering that treatment to the relevant population. Brown et al. (2024) note:

Evidence-based Practice. Incorporation of findings from evidence into practice.

> *Evidence-based practice has over the last decade been marked in its influence within diverse fields...EBP approaches enlist evidence to inform policy making and professional practice. In part EBP*

DOI: 10.4324/9781003431213-22

was a manifestation of scepticism towards the judgement of professionals, the increased availability of data sets and furthering attempts to obtain value for money in public projects.

Brown et al., 2024, pp. 176.

The need for robust EBP has been highlighted throughout this book via examples of where things have gone wrong and which may have been avoided had practice been based on evidence (e.g., Box 11.4); or where research evidence has enhanced practice (e.g., Box 16.1).

Evidence-based practice aims to share **best practice** – particularly given increasing transparency in organisational activities, and with individual practitioners being held to account when things go wrong (e.g., Box 13.1). Simultaneously, owing to the high financial costs of crime (see Wickramasekera et al., 2015) and given current austerity with cuts and crises in criminal justice services – 'value for money' is being prioritised worldwide. Ensuring that practitioners are providing best practice with limited resources and utilising appropriate evidence provides justification for activities and spending – for both organisations and individuals.

Best Practice. Accepted procedures as being most effective.

Utilisation of Research in Policy and Practice

Monk and Koziarski (2023) highlight that before application replication of research findings is critical to ensure reliability. They summarise *"scholars should not be putting all their eggs into the baskets of 'originality'"* (p. 519) noting that research is required for knowledge *creation*, but also to *verify* what we think we know. Therefore, while admirable, the drive for increasing educational qualifications in senior staff (e.g., Masters and PhD levels – the latter of which requires innovation and discovery of new ideas) together with enhanced appreciation for impactful research (see Chapter 16), has made essential verification research less appealing, enhancing the risk of policy and practice being based on only partial evidence.

However, as highlighted in Chapter 16, increasingly research is being undertaken in collaboration with, or by practitioners. Such findings are more likely to be implemented as topics are of relevance (Betts, 2022). Also as discussed in relation to research the importance of listening to the 'voice of' criminal justice participants has also been incorporated in policy and practice. Examples include, **victim personal statements** enabling courts to hear the impact of an offence, **restorative justice** giving victims opportunities to communicate with their offender, and ISVA/IDVA (**Independent Sexual/ Domestic Violence Advisers**) services providing victims/survivors with emotional and practical support – such as accompanying them to court. **Family court** hearings increasingly take the views of children into account when making decisions, and the Good Lives Model (see Chapter 15) advocates treatment as a joint endeavour with perpetrators. While there are debates as to specific types and levels of efficacy, such initiatives have generally shown a positive impact providing victims with additional involvement and control over their experiences (Hester & Lilley, 2018; Lens et al., 2015; Shapland et al., 2011) and offenders realising a better life (Willis & Ward, 2013).

Independent Sexual/ Domestic Violence Advisers. Provide victims/survivors emotional and practical support.

Family Court. Hears cases and resolves disputes involving families or children.

The present authors advocate the need for such client-based practice – for example victims of domestic violence may have stayed in their relationships if the abusive behaviour could have been stopped (Harvey et al., 2024). They may not want their partners arrested, or to be moved into a shelter, often in a new area with limited support (particularly if they cannot take their children or pets[1]). As such, proactive school initiatives teaching appropriate behaviour in healthy relationships together with increased financing for community-based **diversion programmes** and initiatives may be more

Diversion Programmes. To prevent or divert from progressing to formal criminal justice – alternative interventions.

beneficial to perpetrators, victims and society than pursuing incarceration via criminal justice. Moreover, when consideration is given to the fact that many abusers are not only repeat offenders (e.g., attack the same victim more than once) but also serial offenders (i.e., may attack different victims – e.g., if their current relationship breaks down) – then such initiatives may also be cost effective. One example is provided in Box 17.1. However, some challenges include a reluctance to fund offender-based initiatives, when victim service funding is severely lacking.

Box 17.1 Applications in real life: Managing perpetrators in the community.

The government Tackling Domestic Abuse Plan aims to "*make sure that those who commit this crime feel the full force of the law*" (HM Government, 2022), yet a recent inspection highlighted a "*lack of focus upon victim safety and poor work with key safeguarding agencies*" (HM Inspectorate of Probation, 2021). Although prevention of offending is a national priority, there is no recommended structure on how this should be done.

In response, a recent example of how perpetrators considered to be 'High Harm' – i.e., have a high likelihood of committing offences which cause harm – are identified, assessed and managed, has been set up by Dorset Police, UK. Its aim is to improve management of individuals who it is believed have committed repeat domestic abuse or sexually harmful behaviours. The intervention aims to enhance public protection, by encouraging behaviour change. Multi-agency panels share information and suggest interventions – for example encouraging individuals to attend courses to reduce violent behaviour, or by disrupting what they do. Perpetrators are tracked and reviewed to consider what works to reduce their offending, or if interventions are unsuccessful, what additional investigative strategies could be deployed to bring them to justice. Initial analysis suggests such strategies are working (Cole et al., in preparation).

Future Challenges

Future challenges include adaptions to pre-existing problems and crimes as well as the emergence of new ones. These challenges necessitate revised topics of research, but also require revisions to practice. For example, those incarcerated may amend their methods of getting drugs into prisons (using drones) necessitating changes to organisational activity (officers searching outside areas; prisons erecting nets). Sex offenders may amend their methods – moving predatory behaviour from the street to online, limiting potential evidence – as outlined in Box 17.2.

Box 17.2   Applications in real life: Differing methods.

Offence 1: A male offender hangs around an area of late-night clubs, approaching many females asking them for a light. One very drunk female obliges and engages in conversation with him. He then rapes her in the street.

Practice would involve obtaining potential evidence from his phone (being in the area for some time); testimony from potential witnesses; CCTV or dashcam evidence; and evidence showing the victim was highly intoxicated and therefore unable to give consent (if this was being used as a potential defence).

Offence 2: An offender joins a dating app, and messages many females. He arranges to meet one for a takeaway coffee in a quiet park close to his address. During their date she needs the toilet, so he invites her into his home where he rapes her.

Practice would involve obtaining evidence of their phone/app contact (arranging a date); his phone being in or around his own home; few potential witnesses, CCTV or dashcam evidence depicting a 'date'; the victim admitting she went into the offender's residence voluntarily. Consensual sexual activity is likely to be used as a potential defence, with limited evidence to the contrary.

In terms of policy, sexual offences have also been reported within virtual reality which poses difficulties in prosecution under current global laws, yet because of their immersive nature can still have significant impact upon a victim (Muslim, 2024; Steffes et al., 2025).

Similarly, organised crime groups have learnt and adapted their offending behaviours. One example is **County Lines drug dealing** (see Stone, 2018) utilising child exploitation such as recruiting 'clean skins' – local youths with no prior criminal record or taking over local homes (cuckooing) rather than risk known drug carriers being stopped and searched. Newer technologies have increased online criminal activity of all kinds, such as **cyberstalking** via apps tracking movements or monitoring social media posts of victims; or adapting old methods to new e.g., drug dealers moving on-street operations to online deliveries, or sex offenders identifying targets online (as in Box 17.2). A continual challenge is to keep abreast of areas of future risk.

County Lines Drug Dealing. Where illegal drugs are transported from one area/county to another. Phone lines used to move/supply the drugs.

Cyberstalking. Use of digital technology to track, harass/threaten an individual or group.

While bringing many benefits, one challenge of having a more diverse society is the broader knowledge required. For instance, some victims of domestic abuse may not be able to divorce their partner owing to cultural beliefs; or increasing the numbers of civilian police staff may impact the nature of training required. Moreover, how to incorporate research knowledge is challenging. Ideally, all those offering support and treatment for domestic abuse cases would have an in depth knowledge of post separation abuse and **narcissistic traits** that perpetrators may use which could impact on their practice.However, practicalities of determining how much knowledge

Narcissistic Traits. Need admiration, grandiosity/self-importance, lack of empathy, entitled, exploitative, arrogant.

is required is difficult. Increasing staff and additional training may bring its own challenges – e.g., the Police uplift scheme (see Chapter 16) has potentially brought additional problems with staff retention (see further reading).

The Way Forward

In navigating a way forward, criminal justice agencies are increasingly allowing themselves to be open to scrutiny and testing. Supervision, reflective practice, and peer reviewing are increasingly common in practice guidance (e.g., Aurora Mawren & Fullam, 2024; Hunt et al., 2024; Part 3 of the National Police Chief's Council Major Crime Investigation Manual) and via academic evaluation (e.g., Sigurdardóttir et al., 2024). Suggestions of how to improve professional forensic psychology practice are also increasing (e.g., Thompson & Frumkin, 2023), as are evaluations and suggestions for improvement to operational services and tools (e.g., Belur et al., 2021; Hadfield et al., 2021).

In the ever-changing environment, continual professional development of staff is essential, and consideration of diversity and cultural influences should be included (Bergkamp et al., 2023). Much of our knowledge base has been drawn from research in the western world, hence there are calls for the consideration of international differences, and collaborations on subjects such as human rights (see Brown, 2024). Moreover, as well as practice, training should also be evidence based upon up-to-date research and delivered by those with appropriate expertise or lived experiences. Knowledge drawn from education – of different learning styles and techniques, should be incorporated, with utilisation of external educational providers where appropriate. As such increasing bi-directional collaboration with universities is encouraged – and reciprocal arrangements could be made. Practitioners giving guest talks and advice to students, and academics giving guest lectures to practitioners or engaging students in applied research are some ways the present authors have sought to encourage this.

The benefits of multidisciplinary collaboration have been acknowledged – however the focus has traditionally been on related areas of research – criminology, healthcare and law. However, broader interdisciplinary working may now be required – e.g., closer engagement with neuroscience and **forensic neurology** for deeper understanding of brain behaviour (see Darby et al., 2024); or collaboration with computer science to consider the increasing capabilities of **machine learning** and **algorithms** to enhance prioritisation of resources for instance (see Belur et al., 2021; Mandalapu et al., 2023).

Forensic Neurology. Applies neurological (nervous system – e.g., brain) expertise to respond to legal questions e.g., competency to stand trial.

Machine Learning. When computers use data to learn/improve without specific programming.

Algorithms. Set of instructions a computer follows to solve a task/problem.

Such collaboration should also enhance the impact forensic and investigative psychology has on policy and practice development. Liaison with government and National/International organisations is key. For example, psychology can consider ways of reducing biases throughout criminal justice, from analysis of witness, investigation of suspects, inferences made in court and assessments in relation to disposal, treatment and release of offenders. We also need to advocate reform – for instance if evidence suggests that the community diversion programmes discussed above may be accepted by victims and be more successful than incarceration, these programmes should be developed and receive adequate, and continued funding.

Summary

Public safety should be the main concern of criminal justice, with wider needs considered by health and other services. Yet forensic and investigative psychologists walk the tightrope between criminal justice and behaviour – helping victims and perpetrators; working with police, in courts, universities, third sector, hospitals, prisons and probation. The variety of remits and roles are increasingly broad. In 1996 Hess predicted forensic psychology *"will be concerned with public policy"* (p. 245), operating within the political arena. Although inroads to both policy and practice have been made, it will be yourselves as readers to ensure this journey continues. We must remain adaptable to current pressures yet true to our ethical and moral obligations – ensuring psychology helps identify, research, embed knowledge, and shares a part in resolving the challenges ahead.

Note

1 Although local authorities have a statutory duty to provide support to victims and their children residing within refuges – places for some e.g., for those with teenage sons are limited.

Further Reading

Websites –Details of criminal justice careers include:
www.joiningthepolice.co.uk/application-process/ways-in-to-policing
www.cps.gov.uk/careers/overview?gad_source=1&gclid=
    EAIaIQobChMI2MSq0PmmiQMVuZNQBh2ovDUyEAAYASAA
    EgJmkfD_BwE&gclsrc=aw.ds
https://prisonandprobationjobs.gov.uk
https://hmctsjobs.co.uk
www.europol.europa.eu; www.eurojust.europa.eu/about-us/jobs
www.icc-cpi.int/jobs; https://unjobs.org/themes/criminal-justice
UK police retention difficulties are described in this blog www.bluel
    ightleavers.com/blog/I-Don%27t-Want%20to-Be-a-Police-Offi
    cer-Anymore#:~:text=Since%202013%2F14%2C%20attrition%20ra
    tes,6.8%25%20for%202022%2F23
Burnout in forensic psychologists is the topic of this thesis
https://digitalcommons.nl.edu/cgi/viewcontent.cgi?article=
    1751&context=diss
Victim personal statements are outlined
www.cps.gov.uk/sites/default/files/documents/legal_guidance/joint-
    agency-guide-victim-personal-statement_0.pdf
Restorative justice is described https://restorativejustice.org.uk/what-
    restorative-justice
Role of ISVA/IDVA https://survivorsnetwork.org.uk/get-help/isva-
    service; https://safelives.org.uk/about-domestic-abuse/domestic-
    abuse-response-in-the-uk
A blog regarding the voice of the child in family court www.familylawp
    artners.co.uk/blog/the-voice-of-the-child

References

Aurora, M., Mawren, D., & Fullam, R. (2024). An exploratory evaluation of the impact and acceptability of a structured reflective practice program piloted with staff in a forensic mental health setting. *International Journal of Forensic Mental Health, 23*(1), 37–48.

Belur, J., Posch, K., Davies, K., Hammocks, D., Bradford, B., & Myhill, A. (2021). Domestic Abuse: Testing the RFGV algorithm. https://discovery.ucl.ac.uk/id/eprint/10137604/7/Final%20Report%20Document%20Complete%20v03.pdf

Bergkamp, J., McIntyre, K. A., & Hauser, M. (2023). An uncomfortable tension: Reconciling the principles of forensic psychology and cultural competency. *Law and Human Behavior, 47*(1), 233.

Betts, P. R. (2022). Governing the silence: The institutionalisation of evidence-based policing in modern Britain. *Justice, Power and Resistance, 5*(1–2), 9–27.

Brown, J. M., Figueiredo, M. S., & Horvath, M. A. (2024). Taking stock; A review of the state of forensic psychology as revealed through an analysis of journal articles 2015–20. *Journal of Forensic Psychology Research and Practice, 24*(2), 170–191.

Cole, T., Khan, A., Hambidge, S., Davies, K., & Horvath, M. (in preparation). *Evaluation of the High Harm Unit in Dorset Police.* STAR funded project.

Darby, R. R., Considine, C., Weinstock, R., & Darby, W. C. (2024). Forensic neurology: a distinct subspecialty at the intersection of neurology, neuroscience and law. *Nature Reviews Neurology, 20*(3), 183–193.

Hadfield, E., Sleath, E., Brown, S., & Holdsworth, E. (2021). A systematic review into the effectiveness of integrated offender management. *Criminology & Criminal Justice, 21*(5), 650–668.

Harvey, O., Cole, T., Levell, J., & Healy, J. (2024). Explorations of attitudes towards accessibility and accessing domestic violence and abuse (DVA) perpetrator support programmes by victim-survivors and perpetrators across five European countries. *Abuse: An International Impact Journal, 5*(1), 26–45.

Hess, A. K. (1996). Celebrating the twentieth anniversary of criminal justice and behavior: The past, present, and future of forensic psychology. *Criminal Justice and Behavior, 23*(1), 236–250.

Hester, M., & Lilley, S. J. (2018). More than support to court: Rape victims and specialist sexual violence services. *International Review of Victimology, 24*(3), 313–328.

HM Government. (2022). Tackling Domestic Abuse Plan. Retrieved January 9, 2025 from https://assets.publishing.service.gov.uk/media/6244219bd3bf7f32b317e8f3/E02735263_Tackling_Domestic_Abuse_CP_639_Accessible.pdf

HM Inspectorate of Probation. (2021). *Integrated Offender Management.* Retrieved January 8, 2025 from www.justiceinspectorates.gov.uk/hmiprobation/research/the-evidence-base-probation/specific-types-of-delivery/integrated-offender-management

Hunt, E., Hodges, H. J., Armstrong, N. E., Anumba, N. M., DeMier, R. L., & Holden, C. E. (2024). Forensic psychology is different: Supervision approaches in forensic assessment. *Journal of Forensic Psychology Research and Practice*, 1–22. https://doi.org/10.1080/24732850.2024.2407347

Lens, K., Pemberton, A., Brans, K., Braeken, J., Bogaerts, S. and Lahlah, E. (2015) Delivering a victim impact statement: Emotionally effective or counter-productive? *European Journal of Criminology, 12*(1), 17–34

Mandalapu, V., Elluri, L., Vyas, P., & Roy, N. (2023). Crime prediction using machine learning and deep learning: A systematic review and future directions. *IEEE Access, 11*, 60153–60170.

Monk, K., & Koziarski, J. (2023). Replicating & reproducing policing research. *Police Practice and Research, 24*(5), 519–522.

Muslim, M. F. M. (2024). Legal construction of criminal prosecution against perpetrators of rape in the metaverse. *Peradaban Hukum Nusantara, 1*(1), 59–74.

Shapland, J., Robinson, G., & Sorsby, A. (2011). *Restorative justice in practice: Evaluating what works for victims and offenders.* Willan.

Sigurdardóttir, T. D., West, A., & Gudjonsson, G. H. (2024). The current role and contribution of 'forensic clinical psychologists'(FCPs) to criminal investigation in the United Kingdom. *Journal of Criminal Psychology, 14*(3), 217–239.

Steffes, B., Zichler, A., Salemi, S., & Schneider, T. (2025). Impact and consequences of sexual offences in the metaverse using the example of virtual rape. *Deviant Behavior*, 1–16.

Stone, N. (2018). Child criminal exploitation: 'County lines', Trafficking and cuckooing. *Youth Justice, 18*(3), 285–293.

Thompson, D. W., & Frumkin, I. (2023). Recommendations for establishing or expanding a successful forensic psychology practice. *Practice Innovations.* www.researchgate.net/profile/David-Thompson-55/publication/368976915_Recommendations_for_establishing_or_expanding_a_successful_forensic_psychology_practice/links/65197 c551e2386049decfb5c/Recommendations-for-Establishing-or-Expanding-a-Successful-Forensic-Psychology-Practice.pdf

Wickramasekera, N., Wright, J., Elsey, H., Murray, J., & Tubeuf, S. (2015). Cost of crime: A systematic review. *Journal of Criminal Justice*, *43*(3), 218–228.

Willis, G. M., & Ward, T. (2013). The good lives model: Does it work? Preliminary evidence. In L. Craig, L. Dixon & T. Gannon (Eds.), *What works in offender rehabilitation: An evidence-based approach to assessment and treatment* (pp. 305–317). Wiley.

Index

Social Identity Model of
    Deindividuation 53–55
Social Learning Theory
    55–56
social psychology 4–5, **4** *see also*
    social theories of crime; social
    interactions and situational
    factors, influence of 52–53
social sciences, definition 3
social theories of crime 51–52;
    Control Theory 57; Differential
    Association Theory 55;
    Excitation Transfer Theory
    56–57; labelling 52–53;
    Routine Activity Theory 58;
    Social Identity Model of
    Deindividuation, and gang

membership 53–55; and social
    influence 52; Social Learning
    Theory, and observational
    learning 55–56; Strain Theory
    57–58; subcultural delinquency
    53–55
sociology, and criminology
    10
Stern, William 15
Strain Theory 57–58

Terman, Lewis 14
Titus, Stephen 118, *119*

Worboys, John 173–74
Wundt, Wilhelm 13
Wuornos, Aileen 41

For Product Safety Concerns and Information please contact our EU
representative GPSR@taylorandfrancis.com
Taylor & Francis Verlag GmbH, Kaufingerstraße 24, 80331 München, Germany

www.ingramcontent.com/pod-product-compliance
Lightning Source LLC
Chambersburg PA
CBHW070323270326
41926CB00017B/3730

* 9 7 8 1 0 3 2 5 5 1 3 8 8 *